£3-
KH
'7/8

Births and Power

Births and Power

Social Change and
the Politics of Reproduction

EDITED BY

W. Penn Handwerker

Westview Press
BOULDER, SAN FRANCISCO, & LONDON

Published in 1990 in the United States of America by Westview Press, Inc., 5500 Central Avenue, Boulder, Colorado 80301, and in the United Kingdom by Westview Press, Inc., 13 Brunswick Centre, London WC1N 1AF, England

Library of Congress Cataloging-in-Publication Data
Births and power: social change and the politics of reproduction/
    edited by W. Penn Handwerker.
    p. cm.
    ISBN 0-8133-7787-0
    1. Human reproduction—Social aspects. 2. Human reproduction—
Political aspects. I. Handwerker, W. Penn.
QP251.B6 1990
306.4'61—dc20   89-77272
                                                                                    CIP

Printed and bound in the United States of America

The paper used in this publication meets the requirements of the American National Standard for Permanence of Paper for Printed Library Materials Z39.48-1984.

10   9   8   7   6   5   4   3   2   1

Contents

1

Politics and Reproduction:
A Window on Social Change

W. Penn Handwerker

The birth of a child is a political event. So is its absence, for any or all of the events that comprise human reproduction may be part of a strategy to acquire or extend power, may create new ties of dependence or may provide a means to break ties of dependence. Governments seek to regulate reproduction in a variety of ways, often without being aware of the political effects of what they do. Power blocs within a society construe reproduction according to their own agendas. The regulatory means they seek may or may not conflict. But power bloc agendas may blind all parties to the interests and goals of the people they seek to regulate. Reproduction may constitute a statement of defiance to political gatekeepers—to parents, as when an adolescent girl becomes pregnant in spite of her parents' wishes; or to national or local governments, as when women have more children than those policymakers deem appropriate, or when they have fewer, as has happened recently in eastern Europe. Reproduction may weaken or strengthen governments. The continuous production of new generations provides resources that governments may use, but it also provides a population that must be fed, clothed and housed. Different sectors of a population may grow at different rates. Differential growth of this kind shifts the basis of political power and may change profoundly the political complexion of a society.

Human reproduction is not often thought of in these terms. Rather, childbirth and the events that surround and follow it usually are construed as biological events which, for parents in our society, tend to be perceived as individually significant and as statements of our individuality; which, for social scientists, may both reflect and affect various social and economic processes. This book makes the point that births are generated by power relationships. Births are individually significant, of course. Births are significant within societies, however, only insofar as they cement or change power relationships.

This book is not about politics narrowly conceived as what goes on within the confines of a formal political system. It is about politics in the generic sense that Harold Lasswell identified when he asked "Who gets what, when, and how?" (1936). This book is thus about power— where it comes from, who has it, how you acquire it, what happens when you do, and what happens when you don't. Power relationships shape the character of social relationships and channel the direction of social change. The authors of the chapters that follow explore relationships between power, human reproduction, and the social relations that reproductive behavior reflects, and may change. In the process, they help us better understand issues like

- why some women have large families and other women have small ones;
- how to reduce high birth rates in Less Developed Countries and high teenage pregnancy rates in countries like the United States;
- the failure of family planning programs;
- the intense public debate about abortion in the United States; and
- why some women act in ways that dramatically increase their risk of AIDS (Acquired Immunodeficiency Syndrome).

We shall also see how shifts in power relationships transform the economic, social, and moral dimensions of human behavior. Power accrues to individuals or organizations to the extent to which they control access to strategic resources. Power relationships thus dictate key properties of human social relationships, including the way in which they are morally evaluated and construed in social interaction. Power inequalities generate hierarchical social relationships in which those with power tend to coerce and exploit the powerless, even if they do so unintentionally or unconsciously. People who are powerless, in turn, use a variety of means to subvert the power of resource gatekeepers. These political dynamics both reflect and generate conflicting models of moral responsibility, and constitute one of the most important driving forces of social change.

What Is Power, Who Has It, and How Can You Get It?

Power is the ability to influence or control the behavior and beliefs of others even without their consent. You know who has power over you—anyone or any organization that influences your ability to get access to the resources that you need to live. So it is with the people you will meet in this book. We shall call the people and organizations with power *gatekeepers,* to highlight their role in resource access. The gatekeepers you will meet in this book include children; women as mothers and wives; men as fathers and husbands; schools and teachers; employers, both public and private; and health care providers—nurses, midwives, physicians, and medical care organizations.

We could use the word *resource* to refer to virtually anything and, if we did, it would become meaningless. I will use the word to refer to the energy and nutrients that are necessary for human life, and to all means (access channels) by which they can be acquired. Thus, *resources* are the foods that provide energy and nutrients. Money, land, labor, education, berries, hoes, nets, cattle, husbands, or friends also may be "resources," depending upon the time and place one analyzes. So may any other thing, behavior, concept, or form of life that facilitates resource access either directly or indirectly.

Any means by which a person can gain access to resources can be thought of as a "channel" to that resource. *Resource access channels* may be sets of activities, a person or people, an organization, or some combination of activities, people, and organizations. For example, the activities that constitute "marriage" or a "wedding" would be a resource access channel if husbands or wives are resources. Access channels to the resource of a job may include the activities that constitute "education," a school organization, or individual teachers, employers, friends, or relatives. Gatekeepers, as indicated earlier, are individuals or organizations that function as resource access channels. Health care providers and health care organizations are gatekeepers because illness, disability and death reduce resource access, or threaten to. Thus, you acquire power when you find a way to serve as a resource channel gatekeeper for other people or organizations.

Perfect Equality

Imagine that everyone has equal access to all resources. Everyone will be equal if this condition holds, of course. What you believed, said, and did could be effectively ignored by everyone else, and what anyone else believed, said, and did would have no necessary impact on you. You would have no *social* constraints on what you believed or how you acted, other than agreements you entered into voluntarily, by mutual consent. There would be no grounds for coercion and exploitation.[1]

The Case for Happy English Marriages

Alan MacFarlane (1986) argues that these conditions have long characterized family relationships in England, at least outside the aristocracy. Indeed, he argues that the English have had a "modern" conjugal family system for more than 600 years, one in which husbands and wives, and parents and children interacted largely on the basis of equality. MacFarlane points out that, as early as 1350, property rights of many kinds were held by individuals, women as well as men, children as well as parents. England exhibited a highly complex, stratified society. However, England's private sector had been relatively competitive and open for centuries, and both encouraged and allowed social mobility.

Couples married by mutual consent. Indeed, ecclesiastical law required that consent.[2] There were no rules that stipulated that one could not marry either above or below one's social position, and people did. Parents could and did object to particular unions, and broke up prospective unions that they did not approve, at least occasionally. But children were not bound by parental wishes and frequently married against those wishes for love or for other reasons. MacFarlane argues that most couples married because they found each other mutually compatible. They married for companionship, to share both the joys and the hardships of life. Wills and diaries provide consistent and graphic evidence that couples shared mutual affection, trust, and respect.

With few exceptions, marriage presupposed the ability to be economically independent. Children were expected to establish a residence independently of their parents when they married, and this meant that marriage could take place only when the couple had been able to obtain a house and had access to some means of earning a living. Both husbands and wives contributed to the accumulation of property required for their marriage.

Children, MacFarlane argues, were not essential to a marriage. Barrenness was an unfortunate condition, but did not constitute grounds for divorce, wife abuse, or anger. Parents could exercise autocratic authority over their young children, and frequently did so. But parents also lost this control once their children became adults. MacFarlane argues that parents did not invest in children because English law granted children property rights that protected them against parental exploitation, unlike children in continental Europe. Children began to work early as domestic servants, apprentices, and wage laborers, and their parents could not garnish their incomes. Moreover, active land and money markets provided investment alternatives. One did not have to rely on children in one's old age because this responsibility was assumed by manors, guilds, and the Church Poor Relief (see, e.g., Hanawalt 1986).

When manors and guilds withered, the State took over their poor relief functions. In any event, parental obligations to children outweighed the obligations that children had to their parents. As children left home to work in the homes of others, their parents hired other children in their turn. Because ownership and property rights were individualized, parents could disinherit children, but children also could disinherit their parents. Consequently, even if these organizations did not serve the elderly poor well, children could not be counted on to take up the slack or to support their elderly parents independently. Children were known to steal their mother's inheritance, to cheat their elderly father, and to send an aged mother out to beg for bread. Husbands commonly made provision for the care of their wives in their wills. Retirement contracts made with children or, more often, with strangers, were commonly used to secure an adequate living in old age.

The Case for Unhappy English Marriages

This picture of equality crumbles when you look closely at the relationships between English women and their husbands, parents, and children.[3] MacFarlane's study relies almost solely on documents that convey men's perspectives and opinions. He shows convincingly that men looked on marriage and the rearing of children as activities that limited their freedom and could reduce their material welfare. Marriage could provide a life companion, but, for men, children were not essential. Both were consumption activities.

This was not true for English women, who could provide important assistance to their children, especially their daughters, well into adulthood. Women were dependent on their husbands for their material well-being during their youth. But they looked to their mothers and children for both emotional and economic support throughout their lives. For women, both marriage and childbearing were investment activities.

Miriam Slater's study of the Verney family correspondence (1984), an extraordinary series of documents that spans several centuries and 12 generations, reveals that 17th-century women of the gentry looked to marriage as their only effective means to maintain or improve their material well-being. Spinsters were a drain on family resources and, family affections notwithstanding, they received from their brothers or fathers as little as the law allowed. This was not a novel development and it was not one restricted to the 17th century. Eileen Power (1975:40–41) reports that a similar pattern existed several centuries previously. Jane Lewis (1984:3) reports that English women continued to equate spinsterhood and social failure as recently as the early twentieth century. As Cicely Hamilton observed (1909), marriage was a woman's trade.

Married women were legally subordinated to their husbands and did not acquire substantive control over their income and property until the late 19th century. English statute legalized wage discrimination on the basis of sex as early as 1388 (Hanawalt 1986:151) and women had few independent employment options. Hanawalt's account of peasant women in late medieval England (1986:141–155) reveals that the primary employment opportunities for unmarried women were domestic service (in an urban center, on a manor, or in the home of a brother) and prostitution. Women's work opportunities were broadened to include textile manufacturing with the industrial revolution of the 18th and 19th centuries. However, the market for female labor could be flooded more easily than the labor markets for men because it was so narrow. Consequently, women's wages not only were subject to legal constraints, they were also subject to significant market constraints (Prior 1985). Hanawalt (1986:151) points out, moreover, that while peasant women of the 14th and 15th centuries "could bring suit on their own, they had no access to magisterial roles and seldom even used attorneys." Women's chances for attaining a relatively satisfactory standard of living by themselves, consequently, were negligible. If ladies could improve their material well-being by marriage, women low in the English social hierarchy were likely to find that marriage improved their livelihood substantially more, at least when they were young. As recently as the late 19th and early 20th centuries, the average wage of such women was below subsistence levels (Lewis 1984:3).

John Burnett (1982) has edited and provided a synthesis of about 800 autobiographies that described what people remembered of their childhood, education, and families over the period from 1820 to 1920. These autobiographies reveal that mothers are remembered as those who were primarily responsible for family maintenance, budgeting, and care of the house and children (also see Lewis 1984). Burnett points out that fathers are remembered all too commonly as "a drunkard, often thoughtless and uncaring of wife and children, bad tempered and selfish, but occasionally over-generous and sentimental" (1982:233). Fathers spent most of their time away from the home drinking with friends and in the company of women other than their wives. When men were home they rarely shared in household chores. They also took the lion's share of the family resources and they abused their wives. More often than not, men alienated their children and wives and were perceived as irresponsible. This was particularly true for the vast majority of the English population, those in the lower levels of the social hierarchy. Consequently, sons adopted a protective role toward their mother from an early age; if necessary, they physically restrained their father during parental arguments. Mothers, by contrast, are remembered as being overburdened with work. Mothers were remembered occasionally as nagging and demanding, and thus not always warmly. But where children developed relationships with their fathers that are generously described as "remote," children developed close emotional relationships with their mothers. Mothers are remembered consistently as performing innumerable, onerous chores without thought of themselves and often at great sacrifice, especially when they were deserted by their husbands.

Thus, it is understandable, as MacFarlane observes, that women were quite anxious to marry and, indeed, that they perceived a great deal of competition for eligible males. For many men, marriage often was very disadvantageous and offered little more than companionship or partnership. On average, men married very late, only in their late 20s, and significant numbers of men never married at all. The age at marriage rose and fell over the centuries with fluctuations in resource access because, for men, marriage was a consumption expenditure for which they had to accumulate sufficient resources.

By contrast, for women marriage was an investment activity and often constituted the only real chance they had to secure a reasonable livelihood. Similarly, men might be interested only marginally in having children, and might indeed come to look upon subsequent pregnancies as merely adding to their burdens. But for women childbearing could secure additional income in their youths and children provided security they otherwise might not have as they grew old.

We know that various means of contraception and abortion were both known and used in England very early. Historical demographic information reveals, however, that fertility control was not widely or effectively practiced and that, within marriage, women bore more than 9 children on average over the course of their reproductive life (Wrigley and Schofield 1983). This was not because husbands wanted large families. To understand why English women bore children throughout their reproductive careers, it is sufficient to observe that without children their lives would have been very bleak indeed.

Power Is Sweet

The English data remind us that power does not have to be wielded like a club to have profound effects. Hierarchical social relationships exist when everyone does not have equal access to resources, as is true in almost all real-life situations. Differences in physical size, qualities of intelligence, knowledge, skills and, perhaps most importantly, the place of individuals and populations in the trajectory of human history, conspire to create inequalities in resource access. Some people and organizations facilitate or impede resource access by others. These gatekeepers have power.

Some writers call the influence that powerful people wield "legitimate" if those who are subject to it believe that the person or organization who wields power is a rightful authority. However, the concept of "legitimacy" is slippery. It is contingent on perceptions and beliefs, and close inspection usually reveals that these vary from person to person and from event to event. Physicians, employers, and governments constitute "legitimate" authorities—but only for some things at some times and for some people. They coerce nonetheless. For social analysis it is most useful to simply call the influence wielded by powerful people or organizations "coercion," whether or not some of the people who are subject to that power believe that they are legitimately coerced from time to time. Moreover, Lord Acton's dictum holds—Power corrupts; absolute power corrupts absolutely. This is not true all the time, nor for all people. As friends of mine in West Africa observe, however, power is "sweet." It tends to intoxicate its holders. Powerful people so regularly act in ways that increase their material well-being at the expense of others that it is fair to say that *any* degree of hierarchy implies a corresponding degree of coercion, corruption, and exploitation.

The effects of power may be subtle, and apparent only in that people who seek access to resources listen to what gatekeepers say, pay attention to what gatekeepers do, and monitor their own behavior, at least in the presence of the gatekeepers. Gatekeepers receive the deference accorded to those who are "influential" (although some resource seekers search for ways to subvert the power of gatekeepers, or to join their ranks). They are the people who are asked to make decisions, give advice, settle disputes, or act as intermediaries.

What Is Sweet for Some Is Bitter for Others

However, the effects of power usually are unpleasant for the powerless. Much of the coercion and exploitation to which women have been subject has centered around their reproductive biology. Women have been subject to clitoridectomies, menstrual taboos that rationalize their exclusion from important social, political, and economic activities, food taboos during pregnancy which commonly reduce the intake of essential nutrients precisely when they are most needed, and treatment as chattels who are important almost solely for their reproductive capacity (and who may be killed, particularly as infants, when that capacity threatens gatekeepers).

Gynecologists and obstetricians are primary offenders in much of today's world. A significant literature has arisen around the offensive and occasionally dangerous treatment that women continue to experience in the hands of physicians trained in conventional Western biomedicine. The abuses to which women continue to be subject run the gamut from being treated as ignorant objects who do not have the sense to understand their own physiological functions to the routine and unnecessary use during birth of episiotomies and cesaerian sections.

Rose Jones' chapter on "The Politics of Reproductive Biology" discusses a phenomenon that is less well-known—corporate exclusionary policies. It has become clear that men and women who are exposed to chemicals in the workplace face increased risks of damage to their reproductive systems. In the absence of clear national guidelines, individual corporations have established their own. These tend to be constructed on the assumption that women are primarily valuable for their reproductive capacity and men are primarily valuable for their work capacity. Typically, these policies exclude working class women from well-paying positions. They are not applied to low-paying positions commonly held by women. Exclusionary policies are designed to benefit the corporation, not its employees, for they justify the failure to institute measures that would make the workplace safe for all.

The irony is that exclusionary policies hold only short-term benefits for the firms that institute them. First, these policies arbitrarily exclude from the pool of eligible workers some who may be the most productive, and, thus, establish constraints on the competitive potential of these firms. Second, these policies threaten the health of the men who are hired for positions from which women have been excluded, and the health of their children. Short-term savings from lawsuits and public relations damage may be negligible compared with the long term cost of health insurance and health care for men and their families. Exclusionary policies thus impair the performance of the U.S. economy as a whole while they threaten the health of all workers and reduce working class women's ability to direct the course of their own lives.

Sweet Pills May Have Unrecognized Bitterness

Coercion exists even when gatekeepers are not aware of their influence. For example, perhaps the last thing that an obstetrician who is trained in the Western biomedical tradition may think of is that his or her handling of pain can change how women experience the process of birth. Yet this is the possibility that Carolyn Sargent raises in her chapter on "The Politics of Birth." Sargent shows that the Bariba of Benin, West Africa, conceptualize pain and painful experiences in terms of honor and shame. The ideal response to pain is stoicism, and Bariba are renowned among outsiders, including the medical personnel who have come to supervise many Bariba births, for their ability to endure excruciating pain without comment.

Bariba women think of childbirth as a display of their own power through an heroic event, and, so, as a means to demonstrate their honor and courage. Within a hospital setting, however, pain is not an acceptable experience; it is one to be managed therapeutically. Bariba women see hospital deliveries as a means to reduce the risk of maternal and child death. The use of Western medical facilities is also a means to improve your standard of living, for it puts you in contact with potential patrons (see Bledsoe's chapter in this volume). Thus, Bariba also see hospitals as a means to facilitate resource access.

Bariba women now look at birth in ways not too differently than they did in the past. But this may be only because the hospitals that they use are inadequately stocked and staffed, and analgesics are rarely approved for women in labor. Elsewhere in the world where hospital deliveries have substituted for home births and where medical management of pain has, consequently, substituted for other methods, women's beliefs about pain and birth have changed profoundly. Sargent points out that the medical management of pain at birth is likely to increase as infrastructural constraints are removed. Once this occurs, Bariba women will not be able to experience the sense of control over themselves that now gives childbirth its distinctive meaning, and they are likely to think about birth in terms very different than they do now.

Children Are a Mother's Joy

Children have been the most consistently and systematically exploited segment of humanity. For some 10,000 years, since the origins of agriculture, children have been a particularly important resource for their seniors—perhaps especially, as the English data suggested, for their mothers. Candice Bradley recently surveyed the work undertaken by children in agricultural communities. She found that children regularly contribute to productive tasks from age 6 on, and that mothers are the primary beneficiaries (Bradley 1987). In most regions of the world, parents have maintained control over their children by functioning as gatekeepers for the strategic resources of land, labor, and the supernatural. Caroline Bledsoe's chapter "The Politics of Children" shows that both biological and foster parents in contemporary Africa, like their counterparts in historical England, also function as gatekeepers for resources that are important in industrial economies—education and jobs, as well as the patrons who can faciliate access to both.

The benefits that children offer their mothers (and, frequently, their fathers) do not wither with the development of an active labor market.

Indeed, the importance of these functions tends to increase as children move into adulthood. For example, Ellen Ross (1986) shows that working class mothers who lived in London in the late 1800s worked their children hard at home when they were young and expected very specific financial returns when their children matured and began to work on their own. Their children looked forward to the day when they could help support their mother, which is not unlike the view taken by many young people in Africa even today. Ross comments (1986:87–88):

> Henry John Begg's formulation of his boyhood dream "to help" might stand for many others: "That was my one prayer, if I could only find some money or get hold of some money to help my mother. Yes. I used to feel so very very sorry for poor old mum you know. Perhaps I'd see her sitting there crying, you know, well, don't know what her trouble was you know." Will Crooks, describing his childhood in the 1850s and 1860s in Poplar, recounts a vivid memory of waking up at night to see his mother crying "through wondering where the next meal is coming from," as she explained. The boy whispered to himself: "Wait till I'm a man! Won't I work for my mother when I'm a man!" Indeed when, at age thirteen, he earned his first half sovereign, he came running home with it: "Mother, mother, I've earned half a sovereign, and all of it myself, and its yours, all yours, every bit yours!" The words of a Pentonville girl, born in 1896 are very similar, yet she was the sixth child, clearly not the first to take a paid job. After working for 3/6d as a "learner" in a garment factory for six months, she finally graduated to better earnings. "Oh—the first—the first time I earned ten bob. Oh I had a little thin—ten shilling piece—wasn't I half pleased when I brought it home to my mum. She gave me sixpence out of it."

Parental well-being has thus depended heavily on the control that parents exercise over their children and on the control a senior generation exercises over its juniors. The relationships between parents and children tend to be marked by clear hierarchy, exploitation, and coercion even in agricultural societies that otherwise exhibit marked egalitarian characteristics. It may have been illegal for English parents to garnish their children's income, as MacFarlane claims, but they did so nonetheless. Burnett's (1982) collection of autobiographies vividly documents parental exploitation of their children, especially through the first half of the 1800s.

Bledsoe's chapter on fosterage shows that that these functions can extend to foster parents as well. Mende women who have many children send some of them to women who have few or none. Neither biological nor foster mothers are indiscriminate either in the children that they send or those that they accept. Children from low-status homes tend to flow to homes of higher status. There they function as servants in return for advantages that were not available in the home into which they were born. Mothers may both accept foster children and foster out some of their own. Why? Foster children are given fewer household resources and, thus, are cheaper to raise. Moreover, such children constitute a potential source of future income and services that extends the fostering mother's support base of her own children. Foster children who move on to a better life may be asked, in turn, to foster one or more of their foster mother's younger children.

Bigger Is Better

What do you suppose happens to a gatekeeper's power if he or she served this function for 10 people? For 50? For 100? Of course, the gatekeeper's power increases.[4] A gatekeeper's power increases with the number of people who seek access to resources through that channel simply because that population constitutes a larger resource fund on which the gatekeeper can draw. Moreover, gatekeepers may experience new opportunities for resource access that did not exist when they could draw upon the resources of only a small number of people.

Thus, gatekeepers commonly prefer large populations and large families. Nathan Keyfitz points out that "As early as the time of Confucius, Chinese writers saw that when the population was too small the land was idle and taxes were not paid. . . ." (1971:41). The book of Genesis calls upon people to increase and multiply. An early Indian manuscript, the *Arthasastra*, observed that population was a source of political, economic, and military strength, "restricted asceticism to the aged, favored the remarriage of widows, [and] opposed taxes so high as to provoke emigration" (1971:42). Similarly, "Roman writers condemned celibacy and advocated monogamous marriage as the type that would produce the most offspring" (1971:42). Tacitus commented that, among the Germanic tribes of northern Europe around 98 A.D., "The larger a man's kin and the greater the number of his relations by marriage, the stronger is his influence when he is old. Childlessness in Germany is not a paying profession" (Tacitus 1948:118). The penalty for childlessness in England was made explicit in 600 A.D. in its earliest law code, that of Aethelbert of Kent, which stipulated that a widow shall inherit one-half of the goods left by her husband, but only if she had born a living child (Briggs 1983:50). Childlessness in contemporary Africa can evoke pity, but it can also evoke witchcraft accusations, community ostracization, and (albeit very rarely) death.

The size of the population of resource seekers continues to be an important issue for gatekeepers in contemporary, industrialized North

America. For example, emigration quotas have long been used to restrict the size of potential voting blocs and interest groups. So may programs that affect births. Martha Ward (this volume) points out that leaders of the black community in Louisiana look at births among their constituents as a source of votes and are suspicious that white-sponsored programs aimed at adolescent pregnancies may be merely a disguised attempt to limit their influence.

Power accrues by census count as well as by voter lists. The 1990 U.S. census will mark the 200th anniversary of the first count. It is also likely to mark the 200th anniversary of recurrent undercounts of people who are among the poorest and least influential in American society (Norman 1989). Thus, it is likely to mark the 200th anniversary of a process that has systematically denied congressional representation, and government services and payments to the people most in need.

The linkage between census counts and political power is not restricted to the United States. John O'Neil and Patricia Kaufert, in their chapter "The Politics of Obstetric Care," show how Canadian physicians acquired monopoly control over childbirth and made midwifery illegal. This has had the effect of taking control over childbirth out of the hands of Inuit communities, and it has reduced the sense of control that Inuit women experience during birth. Home births have been effectively forbidden, and, in recent years, some 60 percent of all pregnant women have been shipped out of their homes in the north to give birth in a remote, southern hospital, without attendance by family and friends. Inuit leaders have become concerned that southern hospital births may not be counted when it comes time to allocate economic benefits to northern communities, and have used the control of obstetric services as a key symbol of their struggle to re-establish some control over local affairs.

Is There Enough to Go Around?

People become anxious when they are not sure if they can get access to the resources that they need, as when resource stocks or flows either rise or fall dramatically, or are very low. As resource access uncertainties increase, people become suspicious. Other people may be secret competitors who will use cooperation to benefit themselves but will not reciprocate. A person who is successful invites jealousy and hostility, and success thus becomes more costly than it would be otherwise. Foresight and planning, like cooperation and reciprocity, have no utility because it is not clear to what end one can realistically plan, or for which cooperation and reciprocity may yield desirable results.

George Foster clearly identified these circumstances and labeled their effects among peasant cultivators as "The Image of Limited Good"

(1967). Peter Wilson identified the same circumstances as having precisely the same effects on the culture of the Caribbean, and he offered a more vivid image—Crab Antics,

> [the] behavior that resembles that of a number of crabs who, having been placed in a barrel, all try to climb out. But as one nears the top, the one below pulls him down in his own effort to climb. Only a particularly strong crab ever climbs out—the rest, in the long run, remain in the same place (1973:58).

Martha Ward describes Crab Antics in her chapter on "Turf and Teens" among the agencies and organizations in Louisiana that vie for federal funding to support programs concerned with adolescent pregnancy. Ostensibly, these groups seek to improve the welfare of disadvantaged young women. Their behavior, however, reveals that they are more interested in defending their respective turf, or in enlarging it at the expense of other groups, than in helping adolescents. Each has its own agenda, and these shape each group's view of "The Problem" of teenage pregnancy in ways that favor it to the detriment of all, adolescent females included. Existing program goals, consequently, are fragmented. No program effectively reaches any adolescent cohort. Not surprisingly, no one has bothered to talk directly with adolescents about the reality that they live in or about what they are really doing. Thus far, no one has even made this suggestion. "None of the professionals," Ward points out, "ever said that the fundamental cause of pregnancy was sperm; no one mentions that the delivery system for sperm is called boys." Similarly, "no one suggested that coercion, through rape or incest, might be a systematic factor in eleven-year-old children getting pregnant," or that contraceptives might not be sufficiently available to couples who want to use them.

Sweetness Is Diluted by Many Drinkers

Competition, which is generated by resource access uncertainties, may benefit no one, as the Louisiana situation suggests. But it can alter the intensity of the coercion, exploitation, and corruption that are implicit in power relationships. The power of gatekeepers rises with increases in the number of people who seek access to resources through a particular channel partly because such increases create resource access uncertainties. Immigrant communities, for example, are commonly subject to hostility and suspicion because they make natives less sure of their continuing ability to maintain their material well-being. Resource seekers may express competition by hostile acts and discrimination. This is the common experience of immigrant or minority groups, but they can act in like ways toward majorities, of course. Resource seekers also can be expected to compete for the attention and favor of gatekeepers. Consequently, to secure access to resources they can be expected to act increasingly deferentially and offer gatekeepers material rewards and services.

Earlier, you were asked what happens to a gatekeeper's power if he or she served that function for as many as 100 people. Turn the question around. What do you suppose happens to a gatekeeper's power if the 100 people who sought access to a particular set of resources could also get access to those resources from 4 other gatekeepers? From 10 other gatekeepers? Of course, the gatekeeper's power decreases.

Resource seekers constitute a resource for gatekeepers because the latter can charge access costs to the former. Gatekeepers' well-being can be maintained at acceptable levels only if they continue to serve gatekeeper functions. By contrast, resource seekers can improve their well-being only if they use the access channel with the lowest resource access cost. Increases in the number of resource access channels generate competition among gatekeepers because they create resource access uncertainties. The creation of new resources or an increase in resources has the same effect. Because gatekeepers who maintain high resource access costs can be by-passed, gatekeepers can be expected to reduce their demands on resource seekers.

The growth of a world economy after 1750 has created increasingly competitive industrial firms and governmental organizations. This has created firms and organizations that have immense power in some areas of social life, but it has also created new opportunities for resource access that have benefitted both women and the children of new generations. England's industrial revolution over the late 1700s and the early 1800s, for example, was accomplished on the basis of legislation that protected infant industries from international competition and that permitted real wages to fall to less than half their level in 1507–08. The maturation of English industrialization was accomplished by providing goods and materials that Germany and the United States used to fuel their own industrial revolutions, by investing in railway development in Latin America and India and so by creating a market for English manufactures and reducing the costs of imported raw materials, and, where possible, as in India and the West Indies, by suppressing industries that might have competed with English firms. Barriers to international competition were brought down in the name of free trade, when English products no longer needed protection. England's industrial economy thus matured as it became increasingly dependent on international trade, which fueled the industrial development of other countries.

By the mid-to-late 1800s, England began to encounter significant economic competition from the United States, Germany, and, by the early 20th century, even from Japan. Both technological changes and competition selected for industrial centralization, the growth of firms with increasingly complex organization, and higher workforce educational requirements. The demands of Empire, made most clear perhaps by the Crimean War debacle, led to the establishment of a system of open, competitive examinations for civil service placement in 1870, just prior to England's greatest imperial expansion over the period 1880 to 1914. Universal education was made compulsory through the primary grades by 1876. Patronage and clientship became more restricted both in the areas of social and economic life to which they could be applied and in the rewards they could accrue. Real wages rose consistently after the mid 1800s. By the late 1800s, the husband-as-breadwinner family model had become an ideal for families throughout the English social hierarchy. The ability to provide for a wife and children had become a key component of a man's reputation. Not having to work had become the mark of respectability for a wife. Improvements in health care brought about a significant reduction in both morbidity and mortality. Women experienced significantly expanded resource access opportunities in an economy and political system that was subject to increasing competition from international sources.

Employment and educational opportunities for women changed radically over this period, and organized feminist movements emerged in the face of men's opposition to women's new resource access opportunities. Women rarely received the pay that men received, women's opportunities for education were much less than men's, women were systematically excluded from the upper echelons of both the public and private sectors, and women's employment was terminated in many fields when they married. But these restrictions were loosened, primarily after 1900, and women worked in increasing numbers nonetheless. Women found employment as unskilled manual labor in a wide range of light manufacturing industries. Far more significantly, women saw an extraordinary growth in employment opportunities as teachers, clerks, shop assistants, and other white collar occupations (Lewis 1984). The civil service doubled in size over the second half of the 19th century and a large proportion of its growth came from the hiring of women. As early as 1854, more than half of all elementary school teachers were women. By 1914, women's employment in this field had increased more than eight times, and women constituted about 75 percent of all elementary school teachers. The Married Women's Property Acts of 1870 and 1882 guaranteed women's rights to property whether it was acquired prior to marriage or afterward, even if they did not succeed in giving married women the legal status of single women.

A Leader Without Followers Has No Power

Clearly, gatekeepers and resource seekers are mutually dependent—gatekeepers can raise resource access costs; other gatekeepers can lower resource access costs; and resource seekers can be expected to seek lower access costs. You can improve or protect your well-being best if you can correctly anticipate the behavior of others, and the best guide to future behavior is past behavior. Information about a person's or organization's behavior can be acquired most accurately and reliably, perhaps, by direct, personal interaction. Personal interaction requires resource expenditures, however, and tends to reduce individual well-being when it is not accompanied by sharing. Thus, the mutual dependence of gatekeepers and resource seekers generates cooperative, personal relationships based on material reciprocities. The exact qualities of these relationships vary in regular ways.

Scratch My Back and I'll Scratch Yours

Cooperative reciprocities assume two things. First, both parties must have resources that they can exchange. Second, both parties must be able to maintain or improve their well-being by participating in the exchange. For example, historically in England retirement contracts appear to have been quite important to men, whose activities tended to alienate their children and who might serve only minor gatekeeper functions for their children. Children fulfilled important labor functions for farmers, craftsmen, and laborers. But, one can argue, the overall importance of these functions was minor for English men. Fathers may have gained some from the labor of their children, but there was an active labor market and the cost of an indentured servant or a hired laborer, whether child or adult, may well have been less than the cost of rearing one—as Bledsoe (this volume) points out as true for the Mende in contemporary West Africa. Men were expected to take care of themselves and were cared for by their children only irregularly. All too often, as Jill Quadagno (1982:150) reports, for men "retirement meant a choice between unemployment and pauperization."

Mothers, by contrast, tended to develop strong emotional ties with their children, for whom they served important gatekeeper functions throughout their childhood and early adult years. Mothers tended to look to their children for critical support in their old age and most children appear to have acknowledged the debt. Grandmother-daughter-grandchildren linkages provided essential family continuity, mutual care, and economic support. Women frequently spent a portion of their early married years living in their mother's home and they took care of their mother when the latter grew old. During the years they lived in separate households, mothers and daughters sought each other's company and support whenever circumstances permitted. Working class mothers who raised respectable daughters who married promising young men raised their own status and economic circumstances along with that of their daughters. Meacham quotes Robert Roberts' account of his own grand-mother,

> widowed early with four children, [she] had the foresight to bypass a mission hall near the alley where she lived and send her three good-looking daughters to a Wesleyan chapel on the edge of a middle-class suburb. Intelligent girls, they did their duty by God and mother, all becoming Sunday school teachers and each in turn marrying well above her station, one a journalist, another a traveller in sugar, and a third a police inspector—an ill-favoured lot, the old lady grumbled, but "you can't have everything" (1977:23).

Sweetness Is Negotiated

Material resources are scarce, however. This means that people cannot engage in reciprocities with all people. On the contrary, they can take part only in a small number of such relationships at any one time. Cooperative reciprocities thus must be selected, and social relationships negotiated.

Cooperation between gatekeepers reduces the resource access uncertainties and competition that stem from increases in resource access channels (C). But such relationships can be important only when the costs of creating and maintaining such ties is low. Hence, cooperative reciprocity among gatekeepers declines as the number of gatekeepers grows. As cooperative reciprocity declines, resource access uncertainties increase. Gatekeepers thus find that they optimize resource access when they compete among themselves, once the number of gatekeepers is large. Gatekeepers who compete among themselves find that it is most advantageous to establish cooperative reciprocities with resource seekers.

All of this is reversed from the perspective of resource seekers, of course. Cooperative reciprocity among resource seekers declines as the number of resource seekers (P) who utilize a particular channel grows, at least when the number of resource access channels (C) remains small. As cooperative reciprocity among resource seekers declines, resource access uncertainties increase. Resource seekers thus find that they optimize resource access when they compete among themselves as their number grows. Resource seekers who compete among themselves find that it is most advantageous to establish cooperative reciprocities with gatekeepers.

Resource seekers find that cooperative reciprocities with gatekeepers are most advantageous precisely when these cross-hierarchical relationships are least advantageous for gatekeepers. Conversely, gatekeepers find that cooperative reciprocities with resource seekers are most advantageous precisely when these relationships are least advantageous for resource seekers.

Hence, the terms of reciprocity change. As the number of gatekeepers (C) grows, resource seekers discover that they can demand increasing levels of resource access for a given cost and that gatekeepers can demand decreasing resource access costs. Conversely, as the number of resource seekers (P) grows when the number of gatekeepers (C) remains small, gatekeepers discover that they can demand increasing levels of resource access (namely, higher resource access costs charged to resource seekers), and that resource seekers must submit to those costs.

This gradient has become enshrined in the anthropological literature as the difference in leadership patterns exhibited by "Big Men" and "Chiefs." Big Men are leaders in small communities where the potential number of gatekeepers (C) is large and the potential number of resource seekers (P) is small. Potential gatekeepers thus must compete with each other to acquire followers, of whom there are not many. Consequently, Big Men have to maintain personal relationships with their followers, they grant followers major concessions, and they have little power. The net flow of resources to Big Men must be positive, if they are to maintain their leadership position, but their profits are marginal. Chiefs, by contrast, are leaders in large communities where the potential number of gatekeepers (C) is small and the potential number of resource seekers (P) is large. Potential chiefs find it most advantageous to cooperate with other potential chiefs, to the detriment of the powerless. Chiefs are not constrained to establish personal relationships with many of their followers, although they may construe their relationships to followers in personal terms (chiefs commonly are conceptualized as "fathers" to their people). Their relationships with followers are marked by clear social distance and deference. The net flow of resources to chiefs includes wives, labor committments, cows, and other goods; their profits are significant. Chiefs thus have significant amounts of power. In some cases, chiefs have immense power.

Sweetness Can Be Calculated

You have seen that resource access costs vary inversely with the ratio of the channels by which individuals can gain access to resources (C) to the population that seeks access to those resources (P). Hence, power is a function of this ratio, K (Handwerker 1989a).

Not all resources are equal, of course. For a particular set of resources, power is a simple function of K. The actual power of an individual or organization, however, is raised or lowered by some coefficient that measures the relative importance of the resources for which they serve as gatekeeper. For example, women's status tends to decline in hunting and gathering societies where men control access to resources that are more important than those controlled by women (Hayden et al. 1986). In either event, however, the power of gatekeepers varies inversely with K; the power of resource seekers varies directly with K. Where K is low, competition is muted and the power of gatekeepers is largely unrestrained. The effect? The well-being of gatekeepers improves at the expense of resource seekers. Where K is relatively high, however, competition among gatekeepers is high, and constrains what they do. The presence of performance constraints reduces the power of gatekeepers, and coercion and exploitation of the people who seek access to resources are relatively minor.

Dependent Women Have Big Families

These relationships explain why some women have large families and others have small ones. For example, parents have power over their children to the extent to which they monopolize the channels by which their children can gain access to resources. If, simultaneously, children occupy positions as resource channel gatekeepers, childbearing will constitute an investment activity.

Under these circumstances, parents can improve or maintain their material well-being only if they maximize fertility or completed family size. Fertility will be largely determined by variables like the proportion of women who are married, the frequency with which couples have sex, and the duration of breastfeeding, not by contraception and abortion. Fertility levels, consequently, will be "high." The exact level of fertility will be determined by such things as variations in women's nutrition and work loads, marriage arrangements, land tenure, and inheritance patterns, which influence more immediate determinants of births like the proportion of women who are married. Constraints imposed by the means people use to access resources thus may lead to distinctive levels of fertility even among people who do not intentionally contracept or abort. K is large for parents (who can seek resources through a potentially large number of children) and small for children (who can seek resources only through a small number of parents). Thus, although we can expect that parents and children will have mutual obligations, we can expect that the obligations children have to their parents should take precedence over the obligations parents have to their children.

The varied interests of men and women may overlap, but they never constitute identical sets and women always function as gatekeepers for the resource of children. Women's power relative to men can be expected to rise when children function as important resource channel gatekeepers for both men and women, as in most African societies. Women's power relative to men falls when children function as important resource channel gatekeepers only for women, as in historical England. Thus, high fertility occurs as one effect of the costs that attach to resources and the means that *women* can use to gain access to resources. Child-bearing constitutes an investment activity for women when their material well-being is dependent either directly or indirectly on their children.

Independent Women Have Small Families

Conversely, childbearing becomes a consumption activity when children do not function as important resource channel gatekeepers, as the case of English fathers makes clear. When children do not function as resource channel gatekeepers, parents can optimize resource access only if they sharply restrict their childbearing. Children do not function as resource channel gatekeepers when resource access opportunities increase and become a function of technical skills and competence. Because the parental gatekeeper position would be subject to selection for lower resource access costs, parental demands on their children can be expected to moderate. We can expect that parents and children will continue to have mutual obligations. Because the number of resource access channels increases for children, however, K becomes small for parents (who can expect support from few, if any, of their children) and large for children (who can seek resources from many gatekeepers in addition to their parents). Hence, we can expect that parents will come to believe that childbearing should not take precedence over other activities and that the obligations they have to their children should take precedence over the obligations that their children have to them.

The industrial revolution brought about a transition from very high levels of fertility to ones so low that the births that occur do not replace the people who die. The wisdom of conventional social theory tells us that this transition to below-replacement fertility is the outcome of a broad, complex, and highly interdependent process of modernization. This is not so. Fertility transition comes about as one specific effect of a fundamental transformation of women's power relative to men, their parents, and their children.

In England, the birthplace of the industrial revolution, women's power increased as the world economy grew and created increasingly competitive industrial firms and governmental organizations. Who you were and who you knew became less important than your personal skills and competence, and career opportunities were opened to women as well as men. Fertility did not fall precipitously or uniformly because the structural changes that eliminated children's gatekeeper function for their mothers varied with time and place and by occupational and social position. Rising incomes and new goods and services continued to be accessed best through children for significant sectors of the English population, both urban and rural, well into the early 20th century. Declining levels of infant and early childhood mortality merely improved the economic circumstances of such families. Women in this situation did not limit their fertility or did so only in minor ways.

The English fertility transition began first, some time in the late Victorian period, primarily in the mid-to-upper levels of the social and economic hierarchy. In his *Victorian Values* (1981), J.A. Banks argues that the English marital fertility transition was initiated because some men in the upper middle levels of the social order became concerned with the costs of raising large numbers of children. In the late 19th century, entrance to a career ladder was becoming increasingly dependent on formal education as England began to be transformed into a meritocracy. Increasing amounts of family resources had to be expended on public school and university education to see to it that the sons of upper middle class parents were to maintain the social and economic position into which they had been born. Marital fertility had to be limited to achieve that goal. However, MacFarlane's (1986) study reveals that Banks's claim cannot be right—English men had been concerned with the costs of marriage and childraising for as far back as we have records.

Nonetheless, Banks's argument appears to be correct in its essentials. Women married to men who were pursuing a meritocratic career ladder found, like their husbands, that they could look forward to a financial security that middle and upper class women of earlier generations could not. Resource access through children was severely circumscribed. In part, this was because children had to pass through increasingly longer unproductive periods of formal schooling. In part, this was because, once they began their own careers, children began to find that personal social relationships of patronage and clientship could not be counted on to create marked improvements in their careers. Mothers' resource access through personal relationships created by their children, which is still of vital importance in much of Africa, became decreasingly important in an economy in which competence was becoming the criterion for employment and promotion. This change in the structure of the English economy freed middle and upper class women from dependence for resource access on their children but did not alleviate their dependence on their husbands (see, e.g., Dyhouse 1986). However, as education became an increasingly important criterion for career and income placement and advancement, such women found that they could contribute to the career advancement of their husbands and, thus, to their own standard of living from their youth to their old age, by reducing the number of children they bore.

English fertility began to fall rapidly, however, only after the turn of the century when women, like men, found that they could look forward to genuine careers, even if those careers paid much less than the ones available to men. Women in the upper and upper middle classes found that they could create careers for themselves in the professions. Women in the lower middle classes and in the working classes began to experience the structural changes that had been experienced earlier by women higher in the English social order, for their husbands' incomes rose and their husbands' occupations began to offer career tracks and regular increases in pay. Moreover, these women found that they too could create careers for themselves—for example, in teaching, midwifery, and nursing. Women's employment did more than merely maintain subsistence. Lavinia Church, along with other women teachers (Copelman 1986), found that her own employment generated a rising standard of living.

The proportion of women who worked prior to marriage increased over the early 20th century, as did the relative proportion of women in the formal work force. Marriage and childbearing came to be looked upon very differently. Marriage increasingly became a genuine option for women, not one which was mandatory for their economic well-being. In the presence of rising real incomes, women found it less necessary to work after they were married. Some women in the lower middle class and in lower levels of the social hierarchy relied solely on their husbands for support, as did most women in the upper levels of the English social hierarchy. Worker participation rates for young married women rose consistently over the 20th century nonetheless (Lewis 1984: 150). Increasing proportions of women found that childbearing had ceased to be an investment activity. Childbearing now restricted one's ability to work, either in a factory or to pursue a career, or to secure a satisfactory level of economic well-being from one's husband's income. Fertility fell because childbearing had become a consumption activity.

It is important to emphasize that childbearing was not transformed from an investment activity to a consumption activity in England merely because worker participation rates for women increased. As indicated earlier, nearly all women were productive workers for most of their lives through most of English history. Women's worker participation rates prior to 1800 almost certainly were markedly higher than they were in the early 20th century. Childbearing ceased to be an investment activity because the character of the economy and the character of the work and its remuneration had changed profoundly and had eliminated children's gatekeeper functions for their mothers.

The gatekeeper functions of children were not eliminated because restrictions were placed on the use of child labor or because education was made compulsory. English child labor laws date to 1847 and compulsory education laws date to 1876. As indicated earlier, children retained their gatekeeper functions for their mothers well into the 20th century, at least in some sectors of the English population. These gatekeeper functions were eliminated by the structural changes that marked the maturation of England's industrial economy.

The maturation of the industrial economy was marked by increases in the level of competition to which English firms and the English government was subject. Material well-being for women as well as men became contingent on the criteria of educational accomplishments and competence. The income flows accessible to mothers through their children necessarily and correspondingly diminished. High fertility came to adversely affect the material aspirations of parents for themselves, their children, and/or both. The moral economy of childbearing and parent-child relationships changed, and fertility transition was initiated.

English marital fertility thus declined as English society "modernized" and as mass public education was established. But English fertility did not fall because of a broad and highly interdependent process of "modernization." Fertility decline can be traced specifically to the elimination of the gatekeeping functions of children, which transformed childbearing from an investment to a consumption activity for women. The elimination of the gatekeeping functions of children for their mothers can be traced to very specific changes in the economy—an increasing dependence on international trade in an increasingly competitive environment, legislation that allowed property rights for married women, and the proliferation of educational opportunities for women and for men that led to increasingly well-paying employment for both. Similarly, English fertility did not fall because mass public education was established or because the average level of education rose. Women who began to limit their family size were those who could use education to free themselves from their prior dependence on the gatekeeping functions of their children. Most English women did not experience these changes until long after the establishment of mass public education.

People Stumble into the Future

Social change does not occur because people are prescient or particularly rational when they make decisions. Research on how people actually make decisions reveals that we are not very good rational decision-makers. Normal adults, Richard Schweder observes (1977), do not easily think in terms of the conditional probabilities that are required for such choices, even when appropriate information exists. Thus, we regularly blind ourselves to effective courses of action even when we have at our disposal enough information to identify them, as Barbara Tuchman pointed out in her book *The March of Folly* (1984).

Normal human thinking processes generate an unceasing stream of unexpected, new ideas and new ways of doing things (Handwerker 1989b). We construct new ways to think and act by a process we call "inference." Thus, new ways to think about ourselves and the world we live in constitute guesses about the best way to go about living. These can only arise out of our past experience in a unique life trajectory that is set in circumstances dictated by the historical experience of the society into which we were born. Our accumulated experience biases even our perceptions. Consequently, perhaps the vast majority of these innovations are not very useful, and many constitute errors of varying magnitude. In practice, we make choices that seem to be the best, given our knowledge of the circumstances that exist when we make a choice. Then we try to correct our mistakes. This process creates both chaos and pattern in human affairs. It creates chaos because the perceptions that we make of ourselves and the social world in which we live are continually subject to unexpected change. It creates pattern as the outcome of *selection.*

Paths Are Created Around Big Rocks

We are living beings and thus must eat. It follows that selection must favor any conceptual or behavioral innovation that improves or optimizes resource access, and it will eliminate innovations that interfere with the process of resource acquisition. We differentiate alternatives by their costs. The presence and intensity of selective pressures thus may be measured as resource access cost differentials. Faced with alternatives, we regularly act on the one that optimizes our material well-being— the one by which we gain the most or lose the least—*even when we are not conscious of doing so.*

Selection, which is only one mechanism of social change, does not operate in the absence of such cost differentials. Thus, alternatives that cannot be differentiated in cost are selectively neutral. Neither alternative may reduce or improve your resource access, or both (or all) alternatives may reduce or improve your resource access by equal amounts. You are free to choose among alternatives like these on highly personal, and even whimsical grounds. Indeed, genuine "freedom of choice" exists *only* when you can choose among selectively neutral alternatives.

"Freedom of choice" is constrained when alternatives have cost differences. "Freedom of choice" is an illusion when the cost differences are significant.[5] You have seen that large families enhance parental (especially maternal) material well-being in some situations and that small families have the same effect in others. Women in the former situation may use family planning services, but they don't use birth control to reduce their family size. Instead, they use family planning services to determine why they have difficulty in getting pregnant; they use birth control to avoid pregnancy while they are in school (and stop once they graduate), to resume sexual relationships during periods which, traditionally, required abstinence, or to have 9 children instead of 15. Women in the latter situation do use birth control to reduce their family size even when family planning services are not available.

Family Planning Programs Can't Move the Biggest Rocks

It is widely assumed that family planning programs are essential for reducing the high birth rates in Less Developed Countries and for solving the "problem" of adolescent pregnancy in countries like the United States, and that they achieve these goals, perhaps primarily, by providing women greater freedom of choice. This viewpoint is one of the great myths of our time. It attributes to family planning programs goals that they cannot, and should not be expected to accomplish, while it simultaneously ignores the real development and human rights impact those programs can and do have.

Family planning programs generally attempt to cajole, persuade, or coerce people into adopting the view that "small families are best." To achieve these ends, some programs adopt a service orientation that recognizes that birth control is a means to many ends, only one of which is lower fertility. Birth control is advocated as a means for spacing births and, thus, as a means for improving a woman's health and the health of her children; as a means for increasing spendable income and the amount of money that can be devoted to each child; and as a means for making available new opportunities for families, but especially for women. Of course, these exhortations assume that childbearing is a consumption, not an investment activity. Consequently, they are meaningless to women who are dependent for basic material well-being on their children.

Family planning programs can provide many important services, nonetheless, as is implicit in Martha Ward's chapter on adolescent pregnancy:

- They can distribute birth control technologies to people who want to use them, but who otherwise cannot get them.

- They can provide medical attention that otherwise might not be available.
- They can provide contact with people who can provide encouragement, emotional support, and counseling in ways that respect women's integrity.
- They can offer women means to circumvent the extensions of men's power represented by formal governmental and church organizations.

Barbara Pillsbury's chapter on "The Politics of Family Planning" documents how important such services can be in Bangladesh, one of the most densely populated regions of the world. Few Bangladeshis have an opportunity to be other than farmers in this country where a tiny minority has excluded the vast majority from the richest and most productive land. The circumstances of the poor in rural Bangladesh mean that women's welfare continues to depend on demonstrated childbearing, but that resource stress is so intense that 4 children rather than 6 optimize women's (and family's) resource access. Infanticide has been the most common response to these circumstances elsewhere in the world, and at earlier periods in human history (Scrimshaw 1978). The documented neglect of female infants in contemporary Bangladesh suggests that infanticide is practiced there, albeit in a disguised form. Sterilization, a one-time procedure that prevents all future pregnancies, is very attractive to women who have already produced a large family. This is perhaps especially so given cultural and physical obstacles that make the provision of other means of contraception extremely difficult, and their use very risky. The provision of sterilization services to Bangladeshi women will not make childbearing a consumption activity, and it will not bring about a fertility transition to below-replacement levels. But the provision of these services can immensely improve the material welfare of the vast majority of Bangladeshis in this, one of the world's poorest countries.

Family planning programs can neither create the jobs nor provide the education necessary for the well-paying employment that frees women from dependence on their children, husbands, and parents. Family planning programs thus cannot bring about fertility transition in Less Developed Countries like Bangladesh, and they cannot solve the "problem" of adolescent pregnancy in countries like the United States. Of course, once women experience the changes in power and opportunities that make childbearing a consumption activity, fertility falls to very low (usually below replacement) levels, and it is as hard to raise fertility as it appeared to be to lower it, as Jeanne Simonelli points out in her chapter "Power and Policy in Hungary."

Between a Rock and a Hard Place

Meanwhile, women who are dependent on children and men for their material well-being face a new, life-threatening risk that they can take few effective steps to avoid—AIDS. In her chapter on "The Politics of AIDS, Condoms, and Heterosexual Relations," Caroline Bledsoe explains how the limited opportunities now open to African women channel them into acting in ways that increase their risk of AIDS. "Fertility," Bledsoe reminds us, "remains a paramount value in Africa." African women in the 1980s, like their Barbadian counterparts in the 1950s (see the next section), find that childbearing is virtually the only means that they can use either to secure their future material welfare or to establish the relatively permanent ties to men that improve their immediate material welfare. Even school girls, who do *not* want to become pregnant, often find it prudent to establish a sexual relationship with a man to provide the means to pursue their schooling. School girls may use a variety of means to limit their risk of pregnancy, but they find it almost impossible to take steps that do not increase their risk of AIDS.

Condom use is one step that may dramatically reduce the risk of contracting AIDS. But condom use also prevents pregnancy. Condom use thus denies a man the children that he wants. Consequently, a woman who asks her sexual partner to use condoms conveys the message that she wants to end the relationship. Moreover, a woman who asks for condom use

- accuses her mate of consorting with other women, or
- implicitly admits either that she has AIDS or is habitually exposed to the risk of AIDS, and so
- implicitly admits that she has an outside lover, is promiscuous or, worse, is a prostitute.[6]

All of the implications of condom use dramatically diminish a woman's ability to establish or maintain the stable relationship with a man that is necessary to maintain or improve her material welfare. Even school girls, who might want to ask their partner to use condoms, find it extremely difficult, and frequently impossible, to insist on their use.

The absence of opportunities that generate the power disparities to which African women are subject are not limited to that continent. They identify "underdevelopment" even in the midst of a wealthy country such as the United States, where mobility constraints on the poorest have created an underclass whose opportunities are limited largely to men, who deal in drugs. American women within the underclass may have even more limited options than African women. The effect? As in

Africa, increased risk of AIDS among women, but complicated and exacerbated by drug-dependency, and manifested as babies who are born drug-dependent or with AIDS. The incidence of newborns whose lives were effectively terminated during gestation by AIDS, drugs, or both, is now reaching epidemic proportions in cities such as Los Angeles. The problem, however, is endemic to the underclass.

Paths Are Opened When Rocks Are Moved

Much of this chapter has made the point that selection generates social change when resource access cost differentials change. The intensity of selection, and the rate of social change, is a function of the size of those cost differentials. Fertility transition in England, as in most of Europe and North America, took place over nearly a century because the structural changes in the national economy that opened new resource access opportunities to women had to respond to the growth of the world economy. Fertility transition can take place much more rapidly today—it took place on the island of Barbados in the West Indies in only 20 years (Handwerker 1989a).

Prior to 1960, the Barbadian economy was characterized by an uncompetitive and oligopolistic resource structure the primary effect of which was to allocate opportunities largely on the basis of personal relationships, and these on the basis of sex, class, and color. Childbearing was an investment activity for Barbadian women. In a woman's youth, children legitimated her claims on income from men, although establishing those claims required her subservience. In her middle age, children provided financial support that could make her independent of spousal support and reduced or eliminated her subservience to an autocratic male. In her old age, financial support from children meant the difference between abject poverty and a moderate, or even comfortable, level of living. Between 1955 and 1965, the Barbadian economy underwent a major structural discontinuity marked by decline in the importance of sugar and the ascendancy of industrial manufacturing and tourism. The economic well-being of these sectors was subject to selection on the basis of quality and cost factors set in international markets; they opened up new resource access opportunities for both men and women, and, by the 1980s, Barbadian women came to be independent agents who were able to chart their own course in life in ways that had been denied to their mothers and grandmothers. Children no longer served effectively as resource access channels. Children thus became consumer durables— albeit very special ones—and bearing children became a consumption activity in which women had to choose between children or television sets and videos. Because women have special obligations to their children, once they are born, that can and do take precedence over many (and perhaps all) other consumer choices, it has become morally wrong that *bearing* children itself take precedence over a women's personal goals and dreams. Fertility fell from a high of about 5 births over the course of the reproductive years to about 2 (close to or just under replacement levels) by 1980.

Paths Deepen When Rocks Are in Place

Simonelli's chapter illustrates the counter point that selection generates the absence of social change when resource access cost differentials do not change. When England was beginning its industrial revolution, Hungary was a land-poor agricultural country much like Bangladesh is today, and until the early 1900s it experienced high fertility levels comparable to those experienced by contemporary Less Developed Countries. But many of the rural poor in Hungary, like their counterparts in contemporary Bangladesh, found that resource stress made unlimited high fertility disadvantageous. When attempts to control pregnancies and births failed, infanticide was the solution. Hungary made the transition to below-replacement level fertility with structural change in the national economy, especially after World War II, and effective means of contraception and abortion became widely available. However, the Hungarian government found that below-replacement fertility, which was advantageous to Hungarian women, impeded national economic goals. Government attempts to raise fertility by the use of government subsidies for childbearing have not been successful because they have not made women's material well-being dependent on their children. On the contrary, Hungarian women have found ways to take advantage of government subsidies for childbearing without raising their overall level of fertility.

Path Construction Is Creative

Thus, selection actually constructs relatively advantageous means of acquiring resources. New ideas or ways of acting may occur initially in contexts where their resource access advantage is not apparent. Selection is a creative process because it takes novelties that, in their original context, may have no apparent resource access advantage and places them together in contexts where they do. Selection thus concentrates the conceptual and behavioral innovations that improve or optimize resource access.

Within societies, we see this process of concentration when an innovation made by one person at one time and place is combined with another, which was made by another person at another time and place, into something, perhaps quite different, by a third person at still another time and place. Thus, Torricelli's finding in 1643 that the atmosphere exerts a pressure at sea level approximately equal to that of a thirty-inch column of mercury was concentrated with others to produce the steam engine and the internal combustion engine, foundations of the industrial revolution (Barnett 1961). The process of concentration that we see at work in societies only occurs within the minds of specific individuals, however.

The Right Path Often Is Confused with the Path That You Take

Normal human thinking processes not only generate the universal human tendency to make mistakes, they also generate an equally universal propensity for people to be self-contradictory—to act in ways that contradict our beliefs, and to believe things that contradict our actions. Something about the way in which our brains operate also makes us experience the discomfort that Leon Festinger (1957) called "cognitive dissonance" when we become aware of these contradictions. The process of concentration is sometimes apparent in the minds of individuals as what Festinger referred to as dissonance "reduction." New ideas and ways of acting tend to be matched up in ways that minimize the conflicts and contradictions we experience.

We can minimize conflicts in a variety of ways. For example, we can deny that they exist or withdraw from them (through depression, regression, or fantasy). We can substitute new goals for ones that provoke conflict. We can compartmentalize our belief and behavior system, as when we believe that abortion is wrong and vote for a strong advocate of capital punishment. We can rationalize and find justifications for nearly anything, as when we ground a decision to have an abortion on the belief that we spare a child a miserable future.

This means that if people come to think about the world in different ways that they will change their behavior accordingly, so long as those changes improve or optimize resource access. It also means that if people find that new forms of behavior improve or optimize resource access, they will change the way they think. If you come to believe that abortion is wrong, you may act in ways that are consistent with that view. Of course, these beliefs and behaviors are consistent if they are selectively neutral alternatives that cannot affect your material welfare. Selection favors these beliefs if childbearing is an investment activity for you. Selection also favors these beliefs and behaviors if you were raised in a home where your parents adopted these beliefs and behaviors.

The Rocks You Face Suggest the Right Path

Imagine that you are a woman who was raised in such a home, are now a senior in college, have been accepted by the medical school of your choice, and find yourself pregnant. For you, childbearing is a consumption activity. It is no longer so easy to believe that abortion is an absolute wrong.

The considerations that lead to your decision to have an abortion or not to are almost endless, and vary with the particulars of your life trajectory. What will your parents think of the pregnancy? Can you keep an abortion secret? Can you have something grow within you for 9 months and still offer the child for adoption? Can you handle the emotional effects of an abortion? How can you support yourself, the child, and go to medical school? Can the father help in substantive ways, even if he wants to and you want him to? Is having a child now what you really want to do with your life?

Issues such as these do not exist when women are dependent on childbearing for their material well-being. They have become important social issues only recently, and only in countries where structural economic change has largely freed women from dependency on their children, spouses and parents. These are the circumstances that Catherine Leone describes in her chapter on "The Politics of Parenthood." Middle-class women in the United States have opportunities that did not exist for their grandparents, and that do not exist today for women in much of the world, including the American underclass. For them, as for all women, parenthood is a responsibility. For them, as *only* for women who can make real choices about what to do with their lives, parenthood also raises a question of freedom. Parenthood thus raises the issue of fairness. Decisions to have a child, or to have another, thus hinge on what is believed to be fair—to themselves, to their husbands, and to existing children.

People for whom childbearing is an activity that optimizes their resource access find it convenient to say that abortion is a fundamental wrong, and have done so throughout history as well as in the contemporary United States. People for whom childbearing is a selectively neutral activity may adopt this view and act on it without loss. In the process, however, they deny to others the fundamental right to act in ways that optimize or improve resource access that they act on themselves. They do not have to take responsibility for a child, they do not experience the loss of freedom that the birth of a child entails, and they deny to women the fairness that is central to reproductive decisions in the contemporary United States. Abortion in these circumstances truly is insurrection, as Warren Hern argues in his highly personal chapter on "The Politics of Choice."

The issue is not whether abortion is "right" or "wrong." What is "right" or "wrong" varies with resource access costs and the power relations that resource access cost structures create. Women who decide that abortion is the right choice for them, may nonetheless believe that abortion is "wrong"—merely that that choice is less wrong than not having an abortion. It is the one that is most fair in the circumstances. Abortion may improve or optimize resource access, and commonly does among women in industrialized countries. Thus, the issue is choice. The conflict between pro-choice and pro-life groups is intense because the issue is whether one group can deny to another the fundamental human right to seek a better life.

Selection generates the propensity for people to believe that what they do is morally right. More generally, this means that resource access costs and the power relationships that those costs generate dictate moral issues. The political dynamics through which social change (or its absence) comes about thus both reflect and generate conflicting models of moral responsibility.

Different Strokes for Different Folks

Mutual moral responsibilities are implicit in the cooperative reciprocities in which people engage. Power relationships set by resource access costs shift the balance of those responsibilities, however. Indeed, what makes the exercise of power "legitimate" in some circumstances and not in others is that resource seekers acknowledge a greater moral debt to gatekeepers than gatekeepers have to them. The scope of that debt varies with resource access costs and, thus, with power relationships. Where conditions approach equality, as in the relationships between Big Men and their followers, there is little scope for the legitimate exercise of power. Where conditions do not, as in the relationships between Chiefs and their followers, there is wide scope for the legitimate exercise of power. Overt social conflict occurs when changes in resource access costs shift power relationships and, thus, create conflicting models of moral responsibility.

These conclusions also apply to parent-child relationships. In West Africa, parent-child relationships express a model of moral responsibility in which children's obligations to their parents outweigh the obligations that their parents have to them. The most common reason that people cite to justify the rightness of this view is that "parents give you life." This model of moral responsibility is grounded on the control that

parents exercise over strategic resources, which children can expect to
acquire over their own offspring.

Barbadians concurred with this view in the 1950s. Young Barbadian
women speaking in the 1980s, however, argued, occasionally with some
vehemence, that "I did not ask to be born!" They had thus turned this
moral precept on its head. Obligations to mothers that used to be taken
for granted—"giving was like breathing" an older woman observed—
now is a major source of conflict between mothers who believe that
their children should support them and children who believe that they
don't owe their mothers anything. It is also a major source of conflict
among adult siblings, who quarrel about who should help support their
mother, and in what amounts. The model of moral responsibility expressed
in Barbadian parent-child relationships has been turned on its head,
and parents now talk commonly about a "breakdown" in family life on
the island, because parents can no longer function effectively as resource
channel gatekeepers for their children.

An increase in women's opportunities and power thus creates gen-
erational conflict between parents who adopt the view that childbearing
should be an investment activity and offspring who do not. Daughters
who find that their material well-being no longer depends on their
mothers simultaneously find that the gatekeeper functions their own
children can perform cease to be important. Childbearing is thus transformed from an investment activity to a consumption activity and women
sharply restrict their reproductive careers. Such conflict arose around
the turn of the century in England when mothers tried to restrict their
children from pursuing a secondary education to acquire a foundation
for significant economic and social mobility (Ross 1986:88–90), which
is a phenomenon with parallels among parents in contemporary West
Africa (Handwerker 1986:104).

An increase in women's opportunities and power also creates conflict
between women and men, where men have served as resource gatekeepers
for women, as they did in England. Such conflict generated organized
feminist movements in Victorian England. Jones's chapter argues that
this has been true also in the United States.

Moreover, an increase in personal opportunities reduces the importance
of personal social relationships among resource seekers. Consequently,
such an increase brings about a general de-personalization of social
relationships, and the use of social relationships to justify material
assistance shifts from being morally right to being morally wrong. Such
an increase in personal opportunities thus brings about a revolution in
the ways in which individual women and men, and entire generations,
relate to one another. These are the changes in social relationships and
fertility that characterize the modern world.

On Paths, Rocks, and Future Destinations That You Did Not Know Existed

Social scientists often write as if social relationships consist of fixed rights, powers, and obligations. Plainly, this is misleading. Caroline Bledsoe's chapter on fosterage emphasizes that Mende adults look to children as *potential* sources of support, not infallible ones. Rights and obligations between kin are not fixed. They are potentialities that claimants must activate. People subject to these claims cannot satisfy everyone, some claimants may receive little and no claimant may be entirely satisfied. People must actively *manage* their social relationships, even if they do not think of it in these terms.

This conclusion can be readily generalized, for it identifies the essential political problem—how to manage social relationships in ways that optimize access to resources when no such relationship guarantees resource access. Over any historical sequence we observe conceptual and behavioral innovation, change in environmental conditions, and changes in demographic characteristics. People favor innovations that improve or optimize resource access—namely, innovations that both create and maintain gatekeeper positions and innovations that create new resources and new resource access channels and thus subvert existing gatekeeper positions and power. Analysis reveals conflict between resource gatekeepers and resource seekers when we look closely at social relationships over any historical period. Historical dynamics reflect conflict between gatekeepers who act to consolidate and extend their position and resource seekers who act in their own interests. The interests of resource seekers frequently can best be served by subverting the position of gatekeepers. Characteristically, the outcome of these conflicts (if it is possible to clearly identify an "outcome") is one that was not foreseen by any of the participants.

Social scientists also often write as if social, political, economic, and moral issues were compartmentalized and could be studied effectively in isolation. Plainly, this, too, is misleading. Social change is a political process that is channeled by the constraint unique to living beings— we must eat. Individuals thus must find ways to get access to the resources that provide energy and essential nutrients. Individuals or organizations that control access to resources acquire power. Power relationships generate the properties of social relationships, including the way in which they are morally evaluated and construed in social interaction, by selection.

Changes in resource access costs generate social change through a process that is expressed as a change in moral responsibilities. Moral responsibilities thus reflect historically specific power relationships and means for gaining access to resources. The right to well-paying jobs, and to the education and technical skills that make those jobs accessible, exist as issues only when these are essential for resource access and when power relationships systematically deny these means to some.

Resource access costs change when environmental and demographic conditions change. Resource access costs also can change when individuals create new ways to think about the world and act in it. This means that *you* can generate social change. The complexities of power relationships in the real world mean that it is virtually impossible for any one person to direct the course of events in ways they might want. Nonetheless, virtually no one is completely without power. Your ability to direct the course of events depends on your capacity to devise ways to serve (more effective) gatekeeper functions for other people or organizations.

Notes

Acknowledgments. This chapter has been improved significantly by helpful discussions and criticisms provided by Catherine Leone, Lisa Madden, Laura Todd, Martha Ward, Peter Weil, Kathy West, and Leslie Zondervan-Droz.

1. Of course, idiosyncratic factors having to do with individual life trajectory experiences and personality characteristics may create power differentials between specific individuals or organizations, and lead, consequently to the exploitation, coercion, and corruption implicit in such relationships. Relationships such as these do not contribute to the predictable regularities in social relationships and social change that we analyze in this book; on the contrary, relationships such as these are unpredictable from social theory and can be explained only by reference to the unique historical and life trajectory factors that generate them.

2. In early medieval England, the church accepted as a marriage any mutual promise to marry that was phrased either in the present or the future tense and that was followed by sexual intercourse. However, village-level evaluations were the prime determinant of what constituted a legal marriage and, by the early 1600s, some communities were treating unions that were not followed by a church ceremony, and the progeny of these unions, as illegitimate (Levine and Wrightson 1980). English law was not changed to conform to this opinion until 1753 (Houlbrooke 1983:79). Despite this change in the law, informal marriages were very common among craftsmen and laborers until the end of the 19th century (Gillis 1984, 1985).

3. The data on England discussed in subsequent pages are reported in more detail in Handwerker (1989a).

4. This statement, as with all the theoretical claims in this chapter, should be properly qualified with the phrase "all things being equal." As we add conditions, the observable effects of power relationships change. The effects of several additional conditions are the subject of analyses that you read about

later in this chapter. One of the more important of the additional conditions that are not analyzed in this chapter is the effect of competition among gatekeeper organizations on the power of their constituent members or employees. This topic is dealt with briefly elsewhere (Handwerker 1987, 1989a:36–37).

5. Genuine "freedom of choice" is observed when alternatives cannot be differentiated by the conditional probability with which they are chosen; "freedom of choice" varies from constrained to illusory to the extent that the conditional probabilities associated with alternatives exhibit increasingly large differences.

6. In the United States, where AIDS has been associated so strongly with male homosexuality, a woman who requests condom use also may question her partner's masculinity (Kathy West, personal communication).

References Cited

Banks, J.A. 1981. Victorian Values. London: Routledge & Kegan Paul.

Barnett, Homer G. 1961. The Innovative Process. Kroeber Anthropological Society Papers 25: 1–25.

Bradley, Candice. 1987. Women, Children, and Work. Ph.D. Thesis, University of California, Irvine.

Briggs, Asa. 1983. A Social History of England. New York: Viking Press.

Burnett, John. 1982. Destiny Obscure. Autobiographies of Childhood, Education and Family from the 1820s to the 1920s. New York: Penguin.

Copelman, Dina M. 1986. A New Comradeship between Men and Women: Family, Marriage and London's Women Teachers, 1870–1914. *In* Labour and Love. Jane Lewis, ed. Pp. 175–194. Oxford: Basil Blackwell.

Dyhouse, Carol. 1986. Mothers and Daughters in the Middle-Class Home c. 1870–1914. *In* Labour and Love. Jane Lewis, ed. Oxford: Basil Blackwell.

Festinger, Leon. 1957. Cognitive Dissonance. Stanford: Stanford University Press.

Foster, George. 1967. Tzintzuntzan: Mexican Peasants in a Changing World. Boston: Little, Brown.

Gillis, John R. 1984. Peasant, Plebian, and Proletarian Marriage in Britain, 1600–1900. *In* Proletarianization and Family History. David Levine, ed. Pp. 129–162. New York: Academic Press.

————. 1985. For Better, For Worse. British Marriages, 1600 to the Present. New York: Oxford University Press.

Hamilton, Cicely. 1909. Marriage as a Trade. New York: Moffat, Yard and Company.

Hanawalt, Barbara. 1986. The Ties That Bound. New York: Oxford University Press.

Handwerker, W. Penn. 1986. "Natural Fertility" as a Balance of Choice and Behavioral Effect: Policy Implications for Liberian Farm Households. *In* Culture and Reproduction. W. Penn Handwerker, ed. Pp. 90–111. Boulder: Westview.

————. 1987. Fiscal Corruption and the Moral Economy of Resource Acquisition. Research in Economic Anthropology 9:307–353.

————. 1989a. Women's Power and Social Revolution. Newbury Park, CA: Sage.

———. 1989b. The Origins and Evolution of Culture. American Anthropologist
91: 313–326.

Houlbrooke, Ralph A. 1984. The English Family 1450–1700. London: Longman.

Keyfitz, Nathan. 1971. Population Theory and Doctrine: An Historical Survey.
In Readings in Population, William Petersen, ed. Pp. 41–69. New York:
Macmillan.

Lasswell, Harold G. 1936 [1958]. Politics: Who Gets What, When, How. New
York: Meridian Books.

Levine, David, and Keith Wrightson. 1980. The Social Context of Illegitimacy
in Early Modern England. *In* Bastardy and its Comparative History. Peter
Laslett, Karla Oosterveen, and Richard M. Smith, eds. Pp. 158–175. Cambridge,
MA: Harvard University Press.

Lewis, Jane. 1984. Women in England 1870–1950. Bloomington: Indiana University
Press.

MacFarlane, Alan. 1986. Marriage and Love in England 1300–1840. Oxford: Basil
Blackwell.

Meacham, Standish. 1977. A Life Apart. Cambridge, MA: Harvard University
Press.

Norman, Colin. 1989. Who Should Count in the 1990 Census? Science 243:601–
602.

Power, Eileen. 1975. Medieval Women. Cambridge: Cambridge University Press.

Prior, Mary. 1985. Women and the Urban Economy: Oxford 1500–1800. *In*
Women in English Society 1500–1800. Mary Prior, ed. Pp. 93–117. London:
Methuen & Co.

Quadagno, Jill S. 1982. Aging in Early Industrial Society. New York: Academic
Press

Ross, Ellen. 1986. Labour and Love: Rediscovering London's Working-Class
Mothers, 1870–1918. *In* Labour and Love. Jane Lewis, ed. Pp. 73–98. Oxford:
Basil Blackwell.

Schweder, Richard A. 1977. Likeness and Likelihood in Everyday Thought:
Magical Thinking in Judgements about Personality. Current Anthropology 18:
637–658.

Scrimshaw, Susan C. M. 1978. Infant Mortality and Behavior in the Regulation
of Family Size. Population and Development Review 4: 383–404.

Slater, Miriam. 1984. Family Life in the Seventeenth Century. London: Routledge
& Kegan Paul.

Tacitus. 1948. Tacitus on Britain and Germany. H. Mattingly, transl. Baltimore:
Penguin.

Tuchman, Barbara. 1984. The March of Folly. New York: Knopf.

Wilson, Peter J. 1973. Crab Antics. New Haven: Yale University Press.

Wrigley, E.A., and R.S. Schofield. 1983. English Population History from Family
Reconstitution: Summary Results 1600–1799. Population Studies 37: 157–
184.

2

The Politics of Reproductive Biology: Exclusionary Policies in the United States

Rose Jones

In February 1974, 27 women out of a total of 1,500 employees at St. Joe's Mineral Corporation in Pennsylvania were to be transferred out of the zinc-smelting department into less hazardous areas unless they could prove they were infertile. One woman was sterilized and allowed to remain in the zinc-smelting department; all others were transferred to positions which paid an average of $0.20 per hour less (Hricko 1978:399).

In January 1975, thirty-seven women at the Bunker Hill lead smelter in Idaho were informed that they could no longer work in lead operations because of the potential effects of this chemical on their future children. All fertile women were transferred to positions that the company considered safe: most for less pay and lost seniority (Hricko and Brunt 1976:A40; Randall 1985:263).

In January 1978, all women working in the pigments department at American Cyanamid in West Virginia were transferred to less hazardous and lower paying positions. Five women "chose" sterilization; two others who wished to remain fertile were transferred to jobs as janitors at reduced salaries (Scott 1984; Andrews 1983:22).

A mother of four working for General Motors in the lead storage battery plant, was one of six women informed that they would have to prove they were no longer fertile in order to continue working with lead. She had herself sterilized instead of being transferred to a lower paying position (Hricko 1978:399).

This chapter examines a newly emerging, yet familiar form of sexual discrimination and labor exploitation in the United States—the exclusion of women from male-dominated occupations based on reproductive issues. The cases cited earlier characterize U.S. business's response to reproductive hazards associated with chemical exposure in the workplace.

Although the Occupational Safety and Health Administration (OSHA), the American Civil Liberties Union (ACLU), and the Equal Employment Opportunity Commission (EEOC) have publicly, albeit inconsistently and ineffectively, stated that exclusionary policies are illegal, unsubstantiated and discriminatory, this has not deterred industry from implementing them (Stillman 1978; see Shilling 1985). Since 1975, women between the ages of 18 and 50 have been increasingly prohibited from working in or applying for occupations deemed "inappropriate" or potentially hazardous to them or their offspring (Andrews 1983), although men are subject to the same reproductive risks associated with the very occupations from which women are being barred.

Exclusionary Policies: An Overview

Currently there are over 55,000 chemicals in commercial use, thousands of which are suspected of having toxic properties (Holcomb 1983). Because research on the health hazards that these substances may pose is so recent, only a fraction of them have been adequately tested. We do know that over 20 million Americans are exposed to chemicals at work, many of which are known to cause sterility, miscarriages and birth defects (Holcomb 1983). Although there is more documentation of the dangers faced by women workers, we now also know that chemical exposure can harm the reproductive systems of *both* men and women through genetic, gametoxic, intrauterine and extrauterine effects (Hricko 1978:395; Gold 1981).

For example, lead exposure continues to be at the center of exclusionary policies aimed at women (Randall 1985:268). OSHA, the federal agency responsible for ensuring that workers have a safe workplace by setting standards, conducting inspections, and correcting hazards, has recommended guidelines for lead exposure (Chavkin et al. 1983). OSHA has determined that excessive lead exposure is linked to *both* male and female reproductive disorders. In men, these disorders include reduced sexual drive, impotence, decreased semen count, and sterility. In women, disorders include abnormal ovarian cycles, premature births, menstrual disorders, sterility, spontaneous abortions and stillbirths (Gold 1981). OSHA maintains that

there is no basis whatsoever for the claim that women of childbearing age should be excluded from the workplace in order to protect the fetus or the course of pregnancy. Effective compliance with all aspects of this standard will minimize risk to all persons and should, therefore, insure equal employment for both men and women. There is no evidentiary basis, nor any thing in this final standard, which would form the basis for not hiring workers of either sex in the lead industry (Gold 1981:12).

Thus, the exclusionary policies of both the Bunker Hill Chemical Company and General Motors (cited earlier), as well as other lead-related industries, have the dual impact of both illegitimately removing women from jobs and subjecting the men who are hired for these jobs to continued health-risks.

In addition to lead exposure, radiation and other chemicals, including anti-neoplastic drugs, touenediamine, DES, carbon disulfide, and the pesticides kepone and carbaryl (Hatch 1984: 166), are known to adversely affect men's sperm count, sperm shape, and sperm mobility. High risk occupations for men that are known to result in reproductive disorders include anesthesiology, radiology, pesticide workers, and those exposed to vinyl chloride (Messing 1983:146). Other studies indicate that exposure to some chemicals produces teratogenic effects in men. For example, wives of operating room technicians (who are likely to inhale escaping anesthesia) have a greater incidence of miscarriage and birth defects (Hricko 1978; Andrews 1983). Wives of men who work with vinyl chloride also incur an increased rate of miscarriage (Andrews 1983).

Marvin Legator, a professor of genetic toxicology at the University of Texas Medical Branch and a leading researcher on reproductive hazards associated with chemical exposure, confirms the nondiscriminatory impact of chemical exposure: "The more we study, the more we see how males are vulnerable to the same chemicals as females" (Holcomb 1983:40). Although it is highly likely that the chemicals which harm women's reproductive systems do likewise to men's, confirmatory studies often have not been conducted. Those which are available are ignored by industry executives, who continue to claim that such policies are designed to "protect" women workers and their children since they are exclusively at risk (Hricko 1978, Ricci 1977). Mark Silverstein, a physician who specializes in occupational health issues for the United Auto Workers in Detroit, adopts a more prudent view: "If scientific research reveals that a woman's reproductive health is at risk through occupational exposure to a particular substance, there is no scientific justification for concluding that a male co-worker is not similarly at risk, unless and until hard data proves otherwise" (Scott 1984:183).

Industry claims that exclusionary policies are designed to "protect" women are hollow. Management does not claim that the fetus or a woman's reproductive capacity is at risk in lower paying, female dominated occupations. For example, although lead operations, zinc-smelting and vinyl chloride production are the primary occupation areas from which women are being excluded, these are not the only ones which submit workers to an increase risk of damage to the reproductive system. In spite of the risks, women are not prohibited from lower paying jobs that entail exposure to lead, like pottery manufacturing (Stellman 1977:178). Furthermore, many other occupations are associated with reproductive risks through chemical exposure from which women are not being excluded. These include radiology technician, radiotherapist, nuclear medicine technician, packager of contraceptive pills, printshop worker, dental technician, garment worker, lab technician, beautician, and nurse (Messing 1983:146; Chavkin et al. 1983:108).

Moreover, management has not expressed interest in protecting women or their fetuses from other risks that are known to exist in other occupations. For example, clerical work, in which 33 percent of all women are employed in the United States, involves risk of exposure to the potentially toxic chemicals ozone and methanol from using copying and duplicating machines. Health care workers, 75 percent of whom are women, are regularly exposed to infectious diseases including viral hepatitis, tuberculosis, and herpes simplex (Hricko and Brunt 1976). Laboratory workers, 83 percent of whom are women, are exposed to x-rays, radioactive isotopes, and toxic and carcinogenic substances including aminodiphentle, benzidine, and beta-proplolactole (Hricko and Brunt 1976). As indicated earlier, operating room personnel are at risk for both cancer and spontaneous abortions from anesthetic gases. Dry cleaning and laundry workers, 64 percent of whom are women, incur an increased risk of cancer due to exposure to tetrachloroethylene (Hricko and Brunt 1976). Hairdressers have an increased risk of respiratory disease from inhaling hairsprays and dyes (Waldron 1983:126). Dental assistants are exposed to mercury through the silver amalgam used in dental restoration (Weiksnar 1976). Textile and apparel workers, 46 percent and 81 percent respectively of whom are women, are exposed to an increased risk of severe lung diseases due to constant exposure to raw cotton dust, synthetic fibers, and organic solvents, including dyes, mothproofers, and asbestos (Hricko and Brunt 1976).

Exclusionary policies are being implemented only where working class women are moving into positions that pay well and that were formerly monopolized by men (Chavkin et al. 1983). Exclusionary policies are not being suggested in the industries where women constitute a large section of the workforce because employers would be unable to replace them at the same low rate of pay (Scott 1984).

Industry's Perspective

U.S. businesses have not adopted any uniform or widely accepted guidelines for implementing exclusionary policies. On the contrary, individual companies have devised their own criteria for excluding employees from certain occupational areas. The result has been a plethora of arbitrary policies that are based on sex-biased research (Scott 1984:184).

In general, industry's response to growing evidence that workplaces subject workers to increase health risks range from apathy to denial to rationalization. For example, one fruit grower, when he learned that male workers had become sterile through the use of the chemical pesticide DBCP, suggested that the chemical be used in the future as a form of birth control (Bellin and Rubenstein 1983:96).

Industry's most common response to exclusionary policies, however, has been denial or rationalization. For example, the Corporate Medical Director of E.I. Dupont de Nemours, justifies exclusionary policies by stating that "it is not that the female is unique, but that we are attempting to protect the fetus" (Gold 1981:10). Jack Kendrick, President of the Bunker Hill Chemical Company, claims that women were not excluded from the lead-smelting section of the plant, but rather that they were given a "choice." Responding to allegations that his plant implements biased exclusionary policies, he stated that "If a job in a lead exposure area becomes available and a woman is next in line for that position, she is asked if she is capable of conceiving a child. If the answer is yes, she will not be given the job. . . . Certainly, no one is 'required to be sterilized', and it is hard to believe that any woman would, under these circumstances, have any job-related reason whatsoever to even contemplate sterilization" (Gold 1981:10–11). The American Cyanamid Company informed its workers of the adoption of an exclusionary clause with the following memo: "The company realizes that it is a very personal and private matter whether or not a woman cannot become pregnant because of surgical procedures. It must be pointed out, however, that this very personal matter will no longer be private if you are permitted, and choose, to remain in one of the (restricted) departments listed . . . above" (Scott 1984:186). The sexual practices of male employees are not scrutinized in this manner by employers.

To date, several major firms have adopted exclusionary policies, including Exxon, Monsanto, DuPont, Dow Chemical, Firestone Tire and Rubber, Allied Chemical Corporation, and B.F. Goodrich (Randall 1985:277). Each of these firms has been free to implement its own discretionary polices. For example, DuPont (Wilmington, Delaware), according to a company spokesperson, "generally excludes women of child-bearing potential from areas that involve significant exposure to compounds that are confirmed to be embryo-toxic or teratogenic" (Ricci 1977:34). The company includes several chemicals within this category, including dimethylacetamide, formamide, Freon-22, hexaflouroacetone, ethylenethiourea and lead. General Motors (Detroit) excludes women from areas which are exposed to lead unless they cannot bear children. Exxon Corporation (New York City) claims not to have an exclusionary policy. A company spokesperson, however, commented that "in practice we have shied away from letting women work with benzene and other suspect chemicals" (Ricci 1977:34).

Economic and Political Dimensions

Employers are well aware that severe economic repercussions are likely to result if chemical exposure is linked to birth defects within the workplace. Consequently, many employers prefer to risk a penalty and/or fines for employment discrimination under the Equal Employment Opportunity Act (EEOC), or unsafeworking conditions under the Occupational Safety and Health Act (OSHA), rather than a possible personal injury lawsuit involving chemical exposure through the workplace. One industry spokesperson states this legal and economic dilemma quite succinctly: "We have to make a judgment about whether to go up against OSHA or EEOC. . . . Since there are no guidelines we've decided to exclude women from hazardous work areas and take a chance that we may be charged with discrimination" (Ricci 1977:36). Another spokesperson admits the same concern by acknowledging that a discrimination charge is less expensive than a personal injury suit (Weiksnar 1976:17). Sexual discimination charges also result in less public relations damage. As Stillman points out, "The comparative consequences of a damages lawsuit versus an employment discrimination action must be carefully weighted and considered. For example, the media exposure and adverse publicity arising from a personal injury lawsuit involving an injured child can be far more devastating for a company than publicity about an employee discrimination action" (Stillman 1978:608).

The legal issue of an employer's liability to a fetus is complex and, as yet, unresolved. However, certain trends and implications can be observed in the law that indicate an employer's preference for excluding fertile women and retaining fertile men in the disputed industries. Under current legislative policies, an employer may be liable to a child who is damaged as a result of either the mother or the father's occupational exposure to a mutagen (Stillman 1978). The precedent for this liability lies in the case of *Renslow v. Mennite Hospital* 67Ill.2d 348, (Ill. 1977), in which the Supreme Court of Illinois held that a child, conceived nine years after its mother was negligently transfused with incompatible blood, had a cause of action against the negligent physician and hospital for its permanent neurological damage (Stillman 1978:607).

The Renslow decision that a child has a right to sue for injuries resulting from pre-conception actions is significant for industries in which men and women are exposed to chemicals that are known to adversely affect their reproductive systems, as well as those which produce birth defects in offspring. Further, the Renslow decision permits the accrual of liability over decades so that in most states a minor has two or three years after reaching the age of maturity to initiate a lawsuit (Stillman 1978:607). The amount of money for which an employer is liable thus can increase significantly, making a successful lawsuit very costly.

Employers prefer to discriminate against women rather than men because it is far easier under current laws for a woman to prove negligence than it is for men. Under current laws, for example, any man who alleges that lead exposure in the workplace caused his wife to bear a deformed child would have to first prove paternity to win such a lawsuit (Randall 1985:268). This extra burden of proof makes it difficult to successfully litigate such lawsuits. However, if a female worker bears a child with birth defects, the potential lawsuits are exceedingly costly (Scott 1984; see Hricko 1978).

Employers prefer to discriminate against women rather than clean up the workplace because the immediate costs of the former are so low (Ricci 1977; Hricko 1978). Moreover, since women have only recently entered the industrial workforce in large numbers and have little seniority, they are easily replaced (Scott 1984).

In sum, U.S. businesses have adopted exclusionary policies as an optimization strategy. By embracing a gender-specific policy for chemical exposure in the workplace, businesses are able to minimize potential losses and maximize actual profits. A sexually-dichotomized labor force permits firms to avoid expensive investments in health-reform that would be necessary if all employees were acknowledged to be equally at reproductive risk. Furthermore, firms can suffer major public relations, as well as financial losses, if it can be proven that chemical exposure in the workplace resulted in a birth defect (Stillman 1978; Chavkin et al 1983:108). In this regard, women are more visible than men, and employers see women as more expendable. Many firms choose exclusionary policies over more immediately expensive changes that would eliminate hazardous work environments (Hricko 1978). These firms are not motivated by a concern for women employees or their fetuses. The effect of exclusionary practices is that all employees become expendable.

Historical Perspective

Exclusionary policies are not a new phenomenon in U.S. labor relations. Indeed, women have been systematically barred from selected occupations for over a century, almost from the inception of the industrial economy. The historical record illustrates the conflict between society's desire to regulate women's working conditions via reproductive issues and women's desire to compete for higher paying jobs.

Exclusionary policies can be traced to the latter part of the nineteenth century when male workers, employers and the state began to use "protective legislation" to prohibit women from working in certain occupations because of women's perceived inferior physical status. Certain types of work were thought to jeopardize women's ability to bear children. Protective legislation first became a public issue in the United States during the early 1870s. One of the earliest attempts to implement legislation to "protect" women in the labor force was initiated by the iron molders union in Brooklyn in 1872. The skilled male workers decided that women should be excluded from the foundries because "We feel that the girl or the woman . . . is the future mother of the American boys and girls" (Kessler-Harris 1984:140).

The obvious impetus for this stand was a desire to eliminate women as competitors for foundry jobs. During the late 19th century, however, wage-earning women in factories and mills had a 30 percent higher mortality rate than that of male workers (Kessler-Harris 1984). People began to fear that women who worked in the growing industrial sector of the U.S. economy would be unable to bear healthy children. No one bothered to enquire closely about why, exactly, women industrial employees exhibited such high death rates. Instead, individual states began to implement statutes that limited women's working hours.

By the early 1900s, courts began to uphold the state's right to sustain women's capacity to reproduce. The Pennsylvania Supreme Court upheld paternalistic legislation and established a precedent for limiting and restricting women's roles as workers. The court justified it's decision on the following grounds: "Sex imposes limitations to excessive and long continued physical labor as certainly as does minority. . . . Adult females are a class as distinct as minors, separated by natural conditions from all other laborers, and are so constituted as to be unable to endure physical exertion and exposure to the extent and degree that is not harmful to adult males" (Kessler-Harris 1984:144). Thus, the state had begun to legally define women's role in society as the bearer of future generations.

In 1908, the United States Supreme Court sanctioned the right of the government to intervene in women's work. In the famous *Muller v. Oregon* decision 208 U.S. 412 (1908), the court said:

> That woman's physical structure and the performance of maternal functions place her at a disadvantage in the struggle for subsistence is obvious. This is especially true when the burdens of motherhood are upon her. Even when they are not, by abundant testimony of the medical fraternity

continuance for a long period of time on her feet at work, repeating this from day to day, tends to injurious effects upon the body, and as healthy mothers are essential to vigorous offspring, the physical well-being of woman becomes an object of public interest and care in order to preserve the strength and vigor of the race. . . . Differentiated by these matters from the other sex, she is properly placed in a class by herself, and legislation designed for her protection may be sustained, even when like legislation is not necessary for men, and could not be sustained. It is impossible to close one's eyes to the fact that she still looks to her brother and depends upon him. Even though all restrictions on political, personal, and contractual rights were taken away, and she stood, so far as statutes are concerned, upon an absolutely equal plane with him, it would still be true that she is so constituted that she will rest upon and look to him for protection; that her physical structure and a proper discharge of her maternal function—having in view not merely her own health, but the well being of the race—justify legislation to protect her from the greed as well as the passion of man. The limitations which this statute places upon her contractual powers, upon her right to agree with her employer as to the time she shall labor, are not imposed solely for her benefit, but also largely for the benefit of all (Stellman 1977:37–38).

With this decision, the courts upheld statutory limits on the number of hours a woman could work in a day or week (Kessler-Harris 1984) and it set in motion a deluge of state laws that were designed to exclude women from certain occupations. Although the assumption of the *Muller v. Oregon* decision was based on the social conviction that society needed to "protect" women, in fact, the decision protected men's jobs. Women were excluded from mines, iron mills, saloons, and concert halls. They were prohibited from operating "dangerous" machinery, cleaning machinery in motion, and working in areas with high levels of dust (although the cotton dust in textile mills was not so defined). Women were also banned from operating elevators, serving as messengers, and lifting heavy weights (Kessler-Harris 1984:145).

However, women were neither restricted nor "protected" in low-paying jobs and in fields that had long been dominated by women workers. Nurses were still permitted to work long night shifts, waitresses continued to lift heavy trays, and women were still permitted to clean offices at night (Chavkin et al. 1983:109; Andrews 1983). Telephone operators were exempted from the law so that women operators could work night shifts, but women were excluded from higher-paying telephone crafts.

The list of occupations from which women were excluded was extended during the second period of protective legislation, from 1908 to 1923, when "occupational diseases" began to be recognized. For example, medical studies began to observe that exposure to lead was associated with miscarriages and deformed children; consequently, women were barred from lead-related occupations in order to protect future generations. Occupations associated with benzene, phosphorous, and dust also were closed off to women (Kessler-Harris 1984). In 1921, the Women's Bureau of the Department of Labor was sufficiently concerned at these exclusions that it warned that "It is very possible that under the guise of 'protection' women may be shut out from occupations which are really less harmful to . . . them than much of the tedious heavy work both in the home and in the factory which has long been considered their special province . . ." (Kessler-Harris 1984: 148).

During the third and final period of protective legislation, between 1923 and the 1930s, the issue of chemical exposure in the workplace became more central to exclusionary policies. In 1933, the Metropolitan Life Insurance Company identified 94 poisonous substances used in 900 occupations, including radium, dyes, lead, mercury, carbon monoxide, benzol and dust (Kessler-Harris 1984:152). High paying jobs became even more inaccessible to working class women.

The historical record illustrates the degree to which our society has been concerned with women's role as both worker and mother. Protective legislation was designed to restrict women's access to certain occupations due to the state's vested interest in their ability to produce healthy children. Protective legislation was also used covertly to restrict women from high paying jobs.

The legislation passed during the protective era were declared unconstitutional in the 1960s after the enactment of the Civil Rights Act. Current exclusionary practices represent a resurgence of those nineteenth century views of women (Andrews 1983).

Implications and Trends

Exclusionary policies highlight the power that at least some U.S. firms can exert over their employees. Unchecked power leads to policies that benefit the firm and exploit its employees. Archaic, patriarchal conceptions of women as "child-producers" and of men as "breadwinners" sanctify these policies and preclude a mindful assessment of their implications.

One of the implications of exclusionary policies is that they narrow the market for women's labor. Thus, they reduce women's chances of working and they reduce the average wage of working women. Exclusionary policies imply that working class women are suitable only for marginal positions in the industrial manufacturing sector of the U.S. economy. These women are forced to remain in jobs with low pay and are prohibited from entering positions with higher pay. They may lose their industrial jobs and be forced to seek work in sectors that have a large number of job-seekers, and which, consequently, pay poorly. It has been estimated, for example, that if women of childbearing age could not work in lead-related industries, almost two out of three female applicants for the 1.3 million jobs in these industries would be turned away (Hricko 1978:400). Furthermore, if industry applied exclusionary policies to all hazardous workplaces, as many as 20,000,000 jobs would be closed to women (Andrews 1983:22). Although exclusionary polices are not solely responsible for the disparity between men's and women's earnings, it is clear that such policies support and intensify gender stratification and inequality in the workplace. In turn, the reduction of earning potential in the workplace compromises the position of women in other social and personal relations.

Exclusionary policies arbitarily exclude from the pool of eligible workers some who may be the most productive. Furthermore, these policies threaten the health of not only the men who are hired for positions from which women have been excluded, but also that of their offspring. If we accept the legitimacy of exclusionary policies, we license industry to remove vulnerable workers instead of cleaning up the workplace (Scott 1984). And if we permit exclusionary policies to go unchecked, we invite further employee exploitation and abuse.

For example, in a series of articles published in the New York Times (1980a,b,c), Richard Severo revealed that petrochemical companies such as Dow Chemical and DuPont, both of which already apply exclusionary policies to their women employees, have been quietly testing thousands of workers to determine if any of their genes make them vulnerable to chemicals used in the workplace (Scott 1984). Severo pointed out that DuPont routinely administers pre-employment blood tests to all black applicants in order to determine whether or not they carry the sickle-cell trait, even though there is no evidence that this trait puts the carrier at greater risk than any other chemical worker (Severo 1980b).

Genetic screening of this sort may well be advisable—if the results are made available to the people who are tested, if the results can be meaningfully related to well-designed medical and genetic research, and if the results are not used to exclude people from jobs that they want without their consent. These conditions are not now met. On the contrary, unregulated genetic screening lends itself to the extension of exclusionary policies to ethnic minorities.

Exclusionary policies are not a viable solution to health disorders in the workplace. They merely exploit people who already have little power. Such policies threaten the health of all workers and reduce working class women's ability to direct the course of their own lives. Industry must be carefully and quickly regulated and monitored in order to avert these trends. The irony is that workers are most in need of "protection" from the policies and practices that claim to be "protecting" them.

References Cited

Andrews, Lori B. 1983. Is Your Job Hazardous to Your Health? Parents 58(8):22–28.

Bellin, Judith, and Reva Rubenstein. 1983. Genes and Gender in the Workplace. *In* Genes and Gender IV. Myra Fooden, Susan Gorden and Betty Hughley, eds. Pp. 87–100. New York: Gordian Press.

Chavkin, Wendy, R. Evanoff, Ilene Winkler, and Ginny Reath. 1983. Reproductive Hazards in the Workplace. *In* Genes and Gender IV. Myra Fooden, Susan Gorden and Betty Hughley, eds. Pp. 101–132. New York: Gordian Press.

Gold, Rachel B. 1981. Women Entering Labor Force Draws Attention to Reproductive Hazards for Both Sexes. Family Planning/Population Reporter 10(1):10–13.

Hatch, Maureen. 1984. Mother, Father, Worker: Men and Women and the Reproduction Risks of Work. *In* Double Exposure: Women's Health Hazards on the Job and at Home. Wendy Chavkin, ed. Pp. 161–179. New York: Monthly Review Press.

Holcomb, Betty. 1983. Occupational Health: The Fetus Factor. Ms 11(11):40–42.

Hricko, Andrea. 1978. Social Policy Considerations of Occupational Health Standards: The Example of Lead and Reproductive Effects. Preventive Medicine 7:394–406.

Hricko, Andrea, and Melanie Brunt. 1976. Working For Your Life: A Woman's Guide to Job Health Hazards. Labor Occupational Health Program/Health Research Group.

Kessler-Harris, Alice. 1984. Protection for Women: Trade Unions and Labor Laws. *In* Double Exposure: Women's Health Hazards on the Job and at Home. Wendy Chavkin, ed. Pp. 139–154. New York: Monthly Review Press.

Messing, Karen. 1983. Do Men and Women Have Different Jobs Because of Their Biological Differences? *In* Women and Health: The Politics of Sex in Medicine. Elizabeth Fee, ed. Pp. 139–148. Farmingdale, N.Y.: Baywood Publishing.

Randall, Donna M. 1985. Women in Toxic Environments: A Case Study and Examination of Policy Impact. *In* Women and Work: An Annual Review. L. Larwood, Ann Stromberg and B. Gutek, eds. Pp. 259–281. Beverly Hills, CA: Sage Publications.

Ricci, L. J. 1977. Chemicals Give Birth to Human Reproductive Woes. Chemical Engineering 84(16):30–36.

Scott, Judith A. 1984. Keeping Women in Their Place: Exclusionary Policies and Reproduction. *In* Double Exposure: Women's Health Hazards on the Job and at Home. Wendy Chavkin, ed. Pp. 180–195. New York: Monthly Review Press.

Severo, Richard. 1980a. Genetic Tests by Industry Raise Questions on Rights of Workers, New York Times. February 3:A1.

_____. 1980b. Screening of Blacks by Dupont Sharpens Debate on Gene Tests, New York Times. February 4:A1.

_____. 1980c. Dispute Arises over Dow Studies on Genetic Damage in Workers, New York Times. February 5:A1.

Shilling, Dana. 1985. Redress For Success: Using the Law to Enforce Your Rights as a Woman. New York: Penguin Books.

Stellman, Jeanne M. 1977. Women's Work, Women's Health: Myths and Realities. New York: Pantheon Books.

Stillman, Nina G. 1978. Women in the Workplace: A Legal Perspective. Journal of Occupational Medicine 20(9): 605–609.

Weiksnar, Melissa. 1976. To Hire or Fire: The Case of Women in the Workplace. Technology Review 79(1): 16–18.

Waldron, Ingrid. 1983. Employment and Women's Health: An Analysis of Causal Relationships. *In* Women and Health: The Politics of Sex in Medicine. Elizabeth Fee, ed. Pp. 119–138. Farmingdale, N.Y.: Baywood Publishing Company.

3

The Politics of Obstetric Care: The Inuit Experience

John O'Neil and Patricia A. Kaufert

Inuit in remote communities of the Canadian North have experienced, within the space of three decades, a transition from birth in the context of home and family, to birth under the care of a nurse midwife in a community clinic, to birth under the control of physicians in hospitals in southern Canadian cities. This chapter is concerned with the political aspects of this history. It discusses obstetric policy as one aspect of the penetration of southern institutions and controls into the lives of people living in the Canadian North.

The politics of one woman's birth experience and the politics of Inuit relationships with Western medical institutions and the larger Canadian society are inextricably linked. Personal feelings of alienation during confinement in southern hospitals reflect macro-political negotiations for greater community control over birthing options: namely, the struggle against the system of internal colonialism that has characterized northern Canada (O'Neil, 1988).

The data for the chapter derive from a research project initiated in response to questions about the evacuation of women for childbirth put by Inuit from the Keewatin communities to senior health officials. Their concerns included the loneliness of women confined in southern hospitals for several weeks, the impact of this separation on family well-being, and the implications that an out-of-territory birth certificate might have for cultural survival (O'Neil et al., 1988). A team of health researchers, administrators, clinicians and Inuit leaders came together and held a series of meetings in each community to discuss these problems. The outcome of the meetings was the development of the research project which is now in progress; it includes a detailed medical record audit and a prospective survey of Inuit women's experience of pregnancy and birth.

This chapter explores the historical and political background to the changes in obstetric policies which have taken place in the Keewatin over the past fifteen years. It uses archival data, government reports and statistics on the place of birth, plus transcripts of the community meetings and material from a series of interviews with physicians, nurses, administrators and Inuit women.

Evacuation for Childbirth

The Keewatin region lies along the western shore of Hudson's Bay and is part of the Northwest Territories. A population of approximately 5,000 Inuit live in an area of 225,000 square miles. There are seven communities lying between 200 and 800 miles north of Churchill and ranging in size from 200 to 1100 people. Churchill itself is 600 miles north of Winnipeg, the site of the nearest tertiary care hospitals. A 30 bed secondary level hospital is located in Churchill and each community has a "Nursing Station". Nursing Stations are best described as outpatient primary health care clinics staffed by one to five nurses, some of whom have training as nurse practitioners or, more rarely to-day, as nurse-midwives.

The annual number of births for all the communities in the Keewatin between 1970–85 ranged from 105 to 161. Routine prenatal care is provided at the nursing stations with most women being seen by a visiting physician at least once or twice during pregnancy. There has been a gradual but steady decline in the number of births in nursing stations between 1971–85 (Kaufert et. al 1987). While a few births still occur in the communities rather than the hospital, these are usually the result of a woman going into labor before the date set for her evacuation south. Official policy no longer supports childbirth in the nursing station as an elective option. Women are sent to either Churchill or Winnipeg two or three weeks before their expected date of confinement with a few leaving much earlier. High risk women are sent to Winnipeg and low risk women to Churchill (only 40% of all births to Keewatin residents in 1986-87 were in Churchill [Gershman, 1987]).

Physicians and health administrators explain the drift towards hospital birth by the efforts of the medical community and government to lower infant mortality and morbidity rates, coupled with the adoption by obstetricians of more and more rigorous definitions of what constitutes risk in childbirth. This explanation strips away and ignores the social, political and historical contexts which are the setting for changes in obstetric policy in the Keewatin. The core argument of this chapter is that the displacement of the traditional Inuit way of birth and the assumption of medical control over childbirth are not isolated phenomena, but part and parcel of the wider history of Northern health care and Northern politics. The nurse-midwife is a pivotal figure in this account, yet her position in the North is also a chapter in another political history, that of midwifery in Canada and the occasional challenge to the medical monopoly over childbirth.

Health, Health Care, and Colonialism

The medicalization of childbirth in the Keewatin is one dimension of the extension of southern power into Northern Canada and of the relationship between illness and colonialism. Any understanding of present policies of obstetric care or of the perception of these policies within the communities must begin with the history of medical care in the Keewatin and the emergence of a Western hegemonic institutional presence into the health arena.

Traditional Inuit ideas about sickness and health have been described as continuous in contrast to the disassociative model of Western bio-medicine (Wenzel 1981). Inuit sought explanations for illness and misfortune in terms of the individual's relationship with his physical, social and spiritual environment. These explanations were both sociological and historical in the sense that misfortune brought about a critical examination of the social order. The healer's role was to facilitate this examination and assist in the construction of new social understandings. The ideology that validated the healer's role and activities emerged through community consensus rather than being imposed to support the interests of a dominant elite.

With the arrival of missionaries and fur traders in most parts of the Canadian Arctic in the 1940s and 50s, illness and health emerged as commodities which could be traded for the spiritual and economic loyalties of the Inuit population. Early missionaries and traders made their meagre medical resources available in exchange for either conversion to Christianity, or monopolistic control over the fur trade. Scheffel's (1983) work in Labrador on the Moravian mission demonstrates clearly that the Moravians selectively withheld medical assistance when members of the surrounding Inuit communities were slow to convert. Gradually, the treatment of illness became a factor in the negotiations surrounding the spiritual and economic orientations of Inuit. This process had a secularizing impact on Inuit understandings about illness and well-being and resulted in less attention being paid to the maintenance of inter-personal codes for social behavior.

Formal western medicine was first introduced in the Canadian North in the 1950s when physicians began to accompany the various ships supplying the missions and trading posts scattered across the Arctic coast (Brett, 1969). The standard response to infectious disease epidemics such as tuberculosis was to remove infected individuals from their communities and relocate them to southern hospitals and sanatoria for extended periods of time. Other options such as encouraging the population to redistribute itself into smaller traditional groups were sometimes proposed by field staff, but were rejected by southern authorities (Lee, 1975; Graham-Cumming, 1969). By separating survivors from their families and dependents, the health care system exacerbated the social damage already incurred as a result of these epidemics and the accompanying high levels of mortality (Hodgson, 1982).

Implicit in this treatment approach was the message that responsibility for decisions regarding the type and location of treatment for diseases was now entirely in the hands of the colonial power. In the name of medical care, government claimed the authority to disrupt family life and traditional patterns of social organization. This demonstration of power had far reaching ramifications in shaping Inuit expectations. Instead of viewing sickness as an event which, with the help of a healer, resulted in increased social harmony and integration, illness was feared not only as a threat to life, but also as a threat to social continuity and autonomy. Sickness facilitated the intrusion of the colonial power into the intimacies of family life and its paternalism was reproduced continuously in the highly emotional context of the medical encounter, the evacuation of the patient, and the breaking apart of families.

The Traditional Way of Birth

In traditional terms, beliefs surrounding childbirth were constructed parallel to general understandings of illness and misfortune. Specific ritual avoidances of particular foods and social contacts were prescribed, and problems in childbirth were regarded as the outcome of a failure to observe these rules. Although shamans were rarely midwives, difficult births sometimes required shamanistic intervention. In the wider context, problems of fertility, the production of males, and infant mortality were all linked to the general sociological framework of standards for interpersonal behaviour.

The risks of traditional childbirth are central to the current debate over childbirth in the North. For governmental and medical authorities, a reduction in infant mortality from the "traditional" (i.e., pre-settlement) period is the justification for all the changes which have been made in obstetric care in the Keewatin. For the Inuit, the belief that "traditional" (i.e. pre-contact) birth was safe is basic to their demand for control over childbirth. The distinction between pre-contact and pre-settlement is an imposed one, for the current discourse blends both periods and reconstructs historical memory to fit ideological needs. The preservation of traditional beliefs in relation to pregnancy and childbirth is part of the re-affirmation of Inuit culture, but it is also a political act. As such, memories of the past are being collected, redefined and shaped to meet the political and symbolic needs of the present community.

The following assertion of the competence of traditional ways is taken from a statement made at one of meetings held in the Keewatin.

> Inuit people do not believe that having a child, being pregnant, birthing is a disease. It's not an illness. It's a way of life, a normal function of a human being. And in the sense that it's not a disease, then they don't think that you absolutely have to be in the hospital. . . . They (the Inuit) have delivered babies before for centuries and centuries.

After talking to older women about their own experience, we found no one model of traditional birthing, in the sense of a set of prescribed procedures which define where birth should be, who should be present or how it should be managed. Certainly, there were traditional midwives, some of whom are still alive. But women also describe births managed by the woman alone; in other cases, they talk about being helped by their husbands or by other women.

> Once one woman found out that someone was in labor, she told other women and they just came to assist because they wanted to. They knew that the woman in labor was scared so they would come to assist.

Systematic differences in birthing traditions between groups among the Inuit have been described in the ethnographic literature (Freeman, 1984: 680; Dufour 1987), but variations in the accounts we have collected so far seem often to be a function of the characteristics of a particular birth or of who was available at a particular time. In this nomadic hunting society, the latter usually depended on the season.

Yet, although there is no single model, certain themes are common to many of these accounts and recurred whenever Inuit women talked to us about childbirth and the past. One is a sense of competence. The emphasis was on personal strength and responsibility. Woman birthed babies in a hastily constructed snow house, or "beside the sled". Often they continued travelling or returned to regular activities shortly after the birth. Their memories reflected a feeling that life was hard, but childbirth was relatively easy and straightforward; a normal event in an otherwise difficult existence.

Managing birth by oneself, or helping other women birth, emerged as a source of pride for women, a public sign of virtue. Competence was linked with the possession of knowledge.

> Back then, the women had the knowledge to take care of a woman in labor . . . we were informed by our elders on what to do and what not to do (Meeting at Rankin Inlet).

Often a comparison was drawn between the present situation in which health professionals claim a monopoly over obstetric knowledge and this traditional time when information about childbirth was disseminated throughout the community, passing from one generation to the next. Another theme is control; the contrast was made between hospital birth, hooked up to machines, and the traditional right of a woman to choose the position in which she would labor.

In these reconstructions of the past, traditional birth is a communal event, rather than an individual and anomic experience in a southern hospital. Whereas hospital birth is disassociated from the community, traditional birth was integrative. Saladin d'Anglure (1984: 494) describes the importance of such relationships in northern Quebec.

> The midwife (sanaji "she who makes") occupied an essential place in the kinship system, as the cultural mother responsible for the role and for settling the sex of the infant (it was believed that male babies could transform themselves into girls at birth, and sometimes the reverse) and for presiding over all the important rites of passage accompanying the first performances of the child, receiving important presents on such occasions. Terms derived from or resembling kinship terms accompanied the relations between the midwife and the children she delivered, and between children delivered by the same midwife; thus uitsiaq "husband-in-law" and nuliatsiaq "wife-in-law" were used reciprocally by a boy and girl with the same midwife.

Participation in birth was the nexus, therefore, of a series of relationships, linking the midwife to the woman she had delivered and to the child. (As a boy grew into a hunter, he would bring part of his "first catch" to his midwife; a girl would give something she had sewn.) The removal of birth out of the community and into the hospital spells the loss of these relationships.

The Nursing Station and the Nurse-Midwife

Infant mortality rates for the Keewatin in the fifties and early sixties are not known, but they were high according to government reports.

These were the years when people were moving from nomadic camps into permanent settlements. Housing conditions were poor, nutrition was deteriorating, and levels of infectious disease were high, particularly tuberculosis. Many of the women giving birth had lived through the periodic famines of the 1950s. The circumstances were unique and the "pre-contact" traditional mortality rate may have been much lower (Fortuine, 1976).

Prior to 1960, Inuit women in the Keewatin could go to the military hospital in Churchill or to a Catholic mission hospital in Chesterfield; most did neither. The annual Report on Health Conditions for the Northwest Territories (1966) estimated that 66% of Inuit births occurred outside hospitals or nursing stations in 1964. (This percentage was calculated on the number of live births known to the authorities; the real figures were probably higher.) "Capturing" childbirth became a critical dimension in the relationships of colonialism and the domination by one society over another.

The first step in the medicalization of childbirth lay in the transfer of births out of the local setting and into the nursing station. Construction of the nursing stations began in 1960 and was completed in 1970. They were staffed by foreign trained nurse-midwives (predominantly British), a group known as the "come-from-aways" in Labrador (Benoit, 1988). They were hired to provide emergency and primary medical care as well as midwifery (O'Neil, 1986; Scott, 1978).

Through their training, professional ties and ideology, the nurse-midwives brought governmental and medical institutions into the communities. The nursing station was government territory and the nurse a government employee. As such, she held a position in a hierarchy which included physicians and administrators working in northern health care and which stretched from the nursing stations to Ottawa. Nurses had to accept and implement directives from higher up the system rather than respond to the demands of the community in which they were working.

Nurses were nonetheless expected to adopt a public health perspective which relied on personal knowledge of individuals and families. This knowledge was often, however, constructed ahistorically and without consideration for broader structural conditions. Labels of "good" and "bad" were based on assessments of personal hygiene, morality and industriousness. These attributes were generally evaluated in terms of an assimilationist model (i.e., in comparison to those Inuit who lived a "White" lifestyle) or a romantic vision of traditionalism with little regard for the conditions of colonialism. Many nurses had little understanding of the tremendous uprooting and readaptation required in the process of resettlement. Nor did they fully appreciate the extremely poor environmental conditions with which women had to cope.

Not understanding Inuit culture, nurses tended to devalue women's roles and functions. This ignorance was sometimes corrected by time and the gradual accumulation of knowledge about the communities in which a nurse worked as a midwife, but only a few nurses stayed longer than a year or two. Turnover was generally high and communities had to continually re-negotiate relationships with new nurses. On the one hand, nurses were often blamed by Inuit for policy issues beyond their influence and control. On the other hand, nurses tended to support medically dominated health policy that contributed to medicalization and southern control of northern health. The occasionally idealized view of the nurse-midwife in the North has to accommodate this notion of the nurse as enforcer of government policy in a community of which she had only limited understanding.

Childbirth and the Nursing Stations

Reminiscences of the very early years suggest that nurses attended births only by invitation, going to wherever the birth was taking place, be it snow house or summer tent. Lee describes her experiences as a nurse in Baffin Island in 1957:

[I] had been alerted to the fact that Oola and Pitsuala were the settlement's two official midwives, but so far had not been asked for obstetrical help. [I] was relieved. [I] worried about faulty hygiene, of course, but felt it wise to leave the Inuit to deal with childbirth as they had always done. The most sensible way of handling the ignorance you've brought to the Arctic, Dorothy, she told herself firmly, is to impose it on others as little as possible (Lee, 1975: 101).

This attitude of respect for traditional ways was soon replaced by the self-assurance of a government convinced it 'knew' what was needed. Mason (1987) quotes from an interview with Otto Schaefer, a physician who worked for the Federal Government in the Canadian Arctic. He described the situation in the late 1960s in the following terms:

There was push from above for more hospital deliveries, and deliveries in nursing stations instead of in tents and igloos. I do not say that I was one hundred per cent convinced that there was a great need for it, but eventually it was inevitable (Mason, 1987: 224).

The pressure was effective; according to the Annual Report on Health in the Northwest Territories for 1968, 97% of births in the Keewatin occurred in a hospital or a nursing station.

The criterion for deciding eligibility for birth in a nursing station in the 1970s was a relatively informal assessment of the likelihood that birth complications might develop. With slight variations, the following statement was included in each of the annual reports from 1969 until 1977 (emphasis added).

> We have continued the policy that see all primagravida and grand multiparae (fifth or subsequent infants) evacuated to a hospital for delivery as are all complicated pregnancies or anticipated complications. Provided no complications ensued at the birth of the first infant or *if all else is well*, second, third or fourth babies are delivered in nursing stations.

Although the criteria for evacuation were not officially changed throughout the 1970s, a gradual and steady decline in the number of nursing station births occurred throughout this period. By the early 1980s, official policy was against any births taking place in the nursing stations.

The community view of the history of these changes is neatly summarized in a comment made at one of the meetings:

> When all the nursing stations moved into our communities, they told us the first child had to be born in the hospital in Churchill or Winnipeg . . . the next five could be born in the settlement . . . every child born after that had to be away to the hospital. Okay, we accepted that. And then what really started this wanting to have children in the settlement was that everybody for any number of children had to go out. There were no more deliveries in town.

Implicit in this statement is a question—why did the shift to hospital birth take place? One set of answers lies in the improvements in transportation which made it easier to plan an evacuation. Better communication systems brought the nurse into closer contact with physicians and administrators to the south and allowed them closer oversight of her work. Changes in obstetric technology increased the apparent gap between nursing station and obstetric ward (Kaufert et al., 1987). But another explanation is that midwifery had few, if any, supporters, except among women and within the communities.

To explain why midwifery in the North went relatively undefended requires a brief digression into the history of midwifery in Canada.

Canada and Midwifery

The nurse-midwives of the Keewatin were working within one of the few countries in the world where midwifery is not legal. Each of the provinces of Canada has a medical act, dating back to some time in the late 19th century, which gives monopoly rights over childbirth to physicians. Medical Services in the Keewatin was a federal government agency and outside provincial jurisdiction, but even so the use of midwives went unchallenged by the medical profession, only because of the special conditions of the North. There was no change in the official attitudes of the profession towards midwifery.

As Biggs (1983) has shown for Ontario, the medical profession worked hard throughout the latter half of the nineteenth century all across Canada to gain control of childbirth and to have midwifery declared illegal. While similar battles were fought in other industrialized countries, the profession achieved monopolistic control over childbirth only in Canada. Mason (1987) suggests that the reason lies in the rural nature of most of Canada which inhibited the development of an organized midwifery resistance movement, such as those which served to protect and sustain midwifery in the more urbanized countries of Europe.

Certainly, Canada was not without midwives or without a demand for their services. Biggs' (1983) work in Ontario and Benoit's (1988) in Newfoundland and Labrador has shown that the "lay" or "granny" midwife was active in the remote rural areas and among the urban poor. Such women had their staunch defenders in the press and in the provincial legislatures, but were powerless against a politically strong and well organized medical profession (Biggs, 1983; Mason, 1987).

While the physicians claimed that the issue was safety, the underlying motivation for the legislation against midwives was economic survival for an over-supply of country doctors (Biggs, 1983; Mason, 1987). At a time when most people relied almost entirely upon their own resources in dealing with illness, birth offered a way for the doctor to gain access to the family. Mason quotes a letter to the Canada Lancet in 1874 in which a physician argues strenuously against an amendment to the Medical Act which would allow provinces to licence midwives:

> Where I am located I have to contend with two of these old bodies and a quack, who I must say have been pretty successful in their attendance, as they get about 60 cases a year, which would amount in my hands to a very decent living for my small family (Mason, 1987, 204).

As Benoit has shown, the "granny" midwives continued to operate among the poor and in the remote rural areas; but the Provincial Medical

Acts effectively prevented the development of formal training programmes or a system of licensing for midwives on the European model. The medical monopoly was occasionally challenged by individual women (such as Lady Aberdeen) and by formally organized groups (such as the Victorian Order of Nurses). For example, in 1910–1911, the V.O.N. promoted a plan modelled on the midwifery training programme in New York, only to have it defeated by an opposition which combined the medical profession and the nursing associations. According to Biggs (1984: 117):

> Efforts to introduce a system of midwifery in Canada were circumscribed by the professional interests of nurses who wished to retain their recently earned professional status and by physicians who wished to protect their financial interests as well as maintain their monopoly over childbirth.

One could say that the irony of the history of midwifery in the north is that the new demands for midwifery services in the south emerged as this enclave of practising midwives started to disappear from the north.

Nurse-Midwifery in the North

The decision to staff the new nursing stations with nurse-midwives has to be seen against this historical background. It explains, for example, why the federal government had to hire abroad. Canadian training programmes did not exist. This history also meant that Canadian physicians, unlike their European counterparts, were not trained alongside midwives. Relationships between the midwives and physicians working in the Keewatin were somewhat eased whenever the latter were British and familiar with midwifery. But the official position of the medical profession was always that the nursing-station was a poor alternative to physician-attended, hospital birth. In the medical view, a midwife managed birth did not count as medically attended.

The Canadian system with its historical rejection of midwifery undoubtedly worked against the survival of the midwife in the North. As described earlier, her ability to function was increasingly circumscribed, as stricter guidelines for justifying a birth in the community were adopted. By the early eighties, none were eligible, regardless of how low a woman's risk status.

For a number of reasons there was no organized opposition to the change in policy among Northern nurses. First, the nurse-midwives who worked in the North were isolated not only in the physical sense, but due to their foreign training, they lacked informal ties which would link them into Canadian nursing networks. Given the Canadian system, they were also without professional colleagues among southern nurses and the status of their midwifery qualification within professional nursing associations was ambiguous.

As policy changed, any nurse midwife who might have regretted the ending of midwifery in the North would have had few natural allies among her nursing colleagues. The midwives working in the North were few in number and had always been a transitory, relatively unorganized, group with a very high turnover. Starting in the mid 1970s, the representation of midwives among northern nurses was diluted as nursing stations were staffed increasingly by Canadian nurses. Then, in the early 1980s a change in immigration policy set restrictions on hiring of nurses abroad, including the nurse midwives for the North.

The Canadian nurses working in the Keewatin in the early 1980s were trained in a medical tradition which said all births should be in hospital. Indeed, the role of the nurse in the community was seen very differently by these new nurses. They were trained in the emerging theoretical paradigms of a school of nursing which emphasized the collaborative role of the health care practitioner in encouraging people to engage in self-help activities (Cardenas and Lucarz, 1985). This training, combined with a more professional attitude (i.e., as contrasted with the missionary motivation of earlier nurses) contributed to conflict between the two nursing traditions in the north. Hence, there was not only a lack of concerted support for midwifery among nurses, but any nurse who still wanted to provide a midwifery service was as likely to be criticized by her colleagues as by the administration.

The demise of midwifery carried costs for the relationships between the nursing station and the community. Seen from the community perspective, the loss of nurse-midwives (and the loss of local birth options) has significantly undermined nurses' roles in northern communities. Nurses' credibility from the community perspective has also suffered. Some loss of confidence in nursing staff is attributable to a community-based perception that nurses who can't deliver babies are not qualified to provide primary health care.

Politics and Childbirth

Obstetric policies in the Keewatin delineate struggle in two arenas; first, the politics of North-South colonial relationships; second, the politics surrounding demands by women for midwifery care in childbirth. For the Inuit, the trend towards southern control over childbirth is considered not only as a hardship for women and their families, but as a threat to long-term cultural identify and survival. These concerns include a persistent worry over children with birth certificates showing they were born outside the Northwest Territories.

> Most of the people are worried that too many of the Inuit children are being born in the district of Manitoba. During the deliberations for Nunavut, they would like to try to settle this so that it could be included in the settlement before anything is done.

> I am worried that if I was born in a place like Coral Harbour and if my baby is born in Churchill, does that mean even though we're same blood, are we considered non-relatives? I am asking this because of the Alaska settlement where anyone born after 1971 was not included in the agreement.

Although assured by various territorial, provincial and federal officials that a Manitoba birth certificate will not affect entitlement to NWT economic benefits, the history of Native-Government relations in North America leaves many Inuit unconvinced. Special status entitlements (as determined by disk numbers, treaty status, band and, in the case of Alaska, corporate enrollments) have played an important historical role in determining eligibility for economic benefits. For many Inuit, the birth certificate issue symbolizes the extent to which these special entitlements have been determined and manipulated by forces external to their communities.

Inuit see the medicalization of birth as a threat to cultural and political autonomy on another level. Concerns range from loss of traditional skills and knowledge, to identity issues, to political entitlement. These concerns are illustrated in the following comment taken from community meetings held in 1986 in various Keewatin communities.

> Nowadays we are told, forget about our Inuit traditional ways. My concern is that when there's a healthy pregnancy, couldn't the mother have her child in her home town with the older Inuit women who have been midwives and with a younger person who has never had experience in delivering babies to help her along, to watch and to observe. Because that would teach the younger generation what our ancestors used to do.

Loss of knowledge is equated with a loss of competence and, therefore, vulnerability; independence lies in regaining control over decision making.

> If the government should suddenly stop giving assistance to the Inuit, where is that going to leave us? We should start doing something about midwives. Should all the assistance be cut back, then at least we would have another alternative to turn to.

Loss of knowledge and the ability to be responsible for oneself is expressed as a sense of profound deprivation in this statement taken from an interview with one of the traditional midwives:

> It's demeaning to a woman to take her rights away, in a sense killing one of the reasons for living, for her purpose was to help with birthing, and birthing was a part of woman's responsibility, and when you take responsibility away from a person, she becomes a worthless person.

This sentiment might also be expressed by those nurse-midwives who would still like to practise in the North, if it were feasible for them to do so.

Clearly, the efforts of nurses (particularly nurse-midwives) to establish themselves as independent practitioners in the Canadian context are threatened by the growing medical control over northern primary health care. It is easy to see the changes in obstetric policy in the North as part of a struggle between nursing and medicine for professional dominance in the primary health care arena. Seen in its historical context, the demise of the Northern midwife is part of a much older competition for control over childbirth between the medical profession, on the one hand, and women and midwives, on the other hand.

The struggle by Inuit for control over childbirth and the struggle for midwifery in Canada have much in common. We suggest that until northern nurses and Inuit see themselves as victims of the same institutional and historical processes, the trend towards medicalization of childbirth, and health in general, will continue to occur.

Acknowledgments

This research was supported by grants from the National Health Research and Development Program (6607-1412-49) and a Health Scholar award to O'Neil (6607-1379-48). The authors are grateful for the assistance of their co-investigators on the project, Drs. B. Postl, M. Moffatt, P. Brown and B. Binns, Ms. Rosemary Brown and particularly our Inuit collaborators, Eva Voisey and Peter Ernerk. However, the conclusions expressed here are those of the authors, and not necessarily shared by our co-investigators. We also thank the people of the Keewatin region for taking the time to discuss the issues described here with us. We are grateful to our Winnipeg and northern research staff, in particular Dr. Penny Gilbert, Ms. Jackie Linklater, Charlotte St. John and Nellie Kusugak, for their assistance.

References Cited

Benoit, Cecilia. 1988. Midwives in Passage: A Case Study of Occupational Change. Ph.D. dissertation (Toronto: University of Toronto).

Biggs, C. Lesley. 1983. The Case of the Missing Midwives: A History of Midwifery in Ontario from 1795–1900. *In* Ontario Historical Society—Ontario History, Vol. LXXV, No. 1.

———. 1984. The Response to Maternal Mortality in Ontario, 1920–1940. Thesis submitted in conformity with the requirements for the degree of Master of Science in the Division of Community Health at the University of Toronto.

Brett, H. 1969. A Synopsis of Northern Medical History. Canadian Medical Association Journal 100:521–525.

Cardenas, B. and J. Lucarz. 1985. Canadian Indian Health Care: A Model for Service. *In* Community Health Nursing in Canada. Stewart et al. (eds.). Toronto: Gage.

Dufour, Rose. 1987. Accoucher Dans un Iglou. *In* Accourcher Autrement. F. Saillant et M. O'Neil, eds. Montreal: Editions Saint Martin.

Fortuine, Robert A. 1976. The Health of Eskimos as Portrayed in the Earliest Written Accounts. Bulletin of the History of Medicine 45:97–114.

Freeman, Milton M.R. 1984. The Grise Fiord Project. *In* Arctic, Handbook of North American Indians. David Damas (ed.). Washington: Smithsonian Institution.

Gershman, Stuart. 1987. Obstetrical Admissions to the Churchill Health Centre of Inuit Women from the Keewatin District, N.W.T.: A Descriptive Analysis. Unpublished manuscript, Department of Community Health Sciences, Faculty of Medicine, University of Manitoba.

Graham-Cumming. 1969. Northern Health Services. Canadian Medical Association Journal 100:526–531.

Hodgson, Corinne. 1982. The Social and Political Implications of Tuberculosis Among Native Canadians. Canadian Review of Sociology and Anthropology 19(4):502–512.

Kaufert, Patricia A., P. Gilbert, J.D. O'Neil, P. Brown, R. Brown, B. Postl, M.M. Moffatt, B. Binns, and L. Harris. 1987. Obstetric Care in the Keewatin: Changes in the Place of Birth 1971-1985. Paper prepared for presentation at 7th International Congress on Circumpolar Health, June 8–12, Umea, Sweden.

Lee, Dorothy. 1975. Lutiapik. Toronto: McClelland and Stewart Limited.

Mason. 1987. A History of Midwifery in Canada. *In* Report of the Task Force on the Implementation of Midwifery in Ontario. Appendix I, Ontario Ministry of Health.

O'Neil, John D. 1986. Health Care in the Central Canadian Arctic: Continuities and Change. *In* Health and Canadian Society: A Sociological Perspective (2nd ed.). D. Coburn et al., (eds.). Toronto: Fitzhenry and Whiteside.

———. 1988. Self-Determination, Medical Ideology and Health Services in Inuit Communities. *In* Northern Communities: The Prospects for Empowerment. Gurston Dacks and Ken Coates (eds.). Edmonton: Boreal Institute for Northern Studies.

O'Neil, John D., P.A. Kaufert, P. Brown, E. Voisey, M.M. Moffatt, B. Postl, R. Brown, and B. Binns. 1987. Inuit Concerns About Obstetric Policy in the Keewatin Region, N.W.T. Paper prepared for presentation at 7th International Congress on Circumpolar Health, June 8–12, 1987, Umea, Sweden.

Report on Health Conditions in the Northwest Territories, 1966. Medical Services, National Health and Welfare Canada, Yellowknife, Northwest Territories.

Saladin D'Anglure, Bernard. 1984. Inuit of Quebec. *In* Arctic, Handbook of North American Indians. David Damas (ed.). Washington: Smithsonian Institution.

Scheffel, David. 1983. Modernization, Mortality, and Christianity in Northern Labrador. Current Anthropology 24(4):523–524.

Scott, Cora L. 1978. Canada's "Barefoot" Midwives. The Canadian Nurse 74(9):41–42.

Wenzel, G. 1981. Inuit Health and the Health Care System: Change and Status quo. Perspectives on Health I 5(1): 7–15.

4

The Politics of Birth: Cultural Dimensions of Pain, Virtue, and Control Among the Bariba of Benin

Carolyn Sargent

In a recent review of the study of therapy management, John Janzen observed that:

> Debate continues regarding the determination of therapeutic decisions, with materialists, hierarchy-of resort advocates, idealists, culture-as-text analysts, transactionalists, and others promoting their views. . . . A focus on the decision-making process in therapy management is able to show how differing paradigms are handled in real life by living actors (1987:80).

In this chapter, I address shifts in paradigms concerning childbirth held by rural and urban Bariba in People's Republic of Benin, West Africa. I suggest that changes in institutional control of childbirth (cf. Feierman 1985) and the increasing influence of an ideology of medical management of obstetrics may contribute to a reformulation of cultural constructs regarding birth. Feierman, in a review article addressing the social determinants of health and health care in Africa over the past century has argued that one of the most difficult and significant puzzles in the study of African healing is who controls the therapeutic process (1985:75). He reiterates that control over healing is important in shaping ideology and that "the struggle to create alternatives illustrates the ideological role of those who control healing" (75).

Correspondingly, I will argue that increasing government control over the practice of obstetrics in Benin, and the concomitant diminishing of the responsibilities of household and lineage with regard to birth, carry implications for the management of birth. As one facet of the argument, I will suggest that Bariba initiation rituals strategically influence the ideology of obstetrics. Government policies regulating such rituals, in turn, are likely to modify Bariba understanding of expected and appropriate behavior for women during delivery. I will focus particularly on concepts of expected behavior in response to pain in Bariba society; the linkages between concepts of pain and therapeutic choice; and the implications of transformations in control of the delivery process for the pain response.

Methodology

The research reported in this chapter was conducted in 1982–83, primarily in Parakou, a town of approximately 60,000 located in northern Benin and includes contextual material obtained in research during 1976–77 in the Bariba village of Pehunko, population 2000. In the Parakou research, I interviewed 123 pregnant Bariba women who attended a prenatal clinic regarding reproductive and family history; 35 pregnant women were interviewed extensively at home concerning reproduction, medical and religious beliefs; and a sample of 50 women employed in a local cashew factory were interviewed to construct a profile of salaried urban Bariba women. In addition, I discussed delivery procedures and behavior with four nurse-midwives staffing the government maternity hospital and with two indigenous urban midwives. Rural data derived from observations of home deliveries, and interviews with 125 women of reproductive age and 18 indigenous midwives.

Agendas for Therapeutic Choice

Research on obstetrical beliefs and practices among rural and urban Bariba has led me to propose that obstetrical decisions are influenced by a complex set of individual goals and priorities, or agendas. These include:

1. *Proverbial virtues*, such as honor, courage, stoicism, typified by Bariba ideals for behavior of both men and women confronted with ordeals in life. For men, the prototypical ordeal falls in the domain of warfare, initiation, or hunting. For women, the major ordeals of life are clitoridectomy and childbirth. The "true" Bariba should face the pain and danger of such ordeals with impassive demeanor and endurance.
2. *Cosmological concerns*, primarily involving witchcraft control. Bariba perceive childbirth as an event with cosmological implications. Because witches may appear at birth, witch detection becomes an integral dimension of delivery.

3. *Status aspirations,* referring to the goal of attaining elite status by success in the civil service or in commerce. This may involve emulation of a so-called "civilized" lifestyle, including European dress, food habits, entertainment and use of government medical facilities.
4. *Medical concerns,* or the search for competent care, leading clients in urban centers to consult an array of indigenous and cosmopolitan practitioners. The marked success of French-sponsored medical campaigns in the colonial period appears to have influenced prospective clients' perceptions of medical competence. In the area of obstetrics, the government strongly recommends hospital delivery. Thus government public health policy and threats of sanctions levied against those delivering at home represent external pressures which affect obstetrical and other medical decisions.

Virtue, Pain, and Obstetrics

Research on childbirth among rural Bariba indicated the predominance of concerns with the "proverbial virtues" described above. Thus ideals of courage and stoicism at delivery are underscored in anecdotes and counsel to young girls and pregnant women and in retrospective accounts of labor and delivery. More broadly, an appropriate response to pain is perceived as fundamental to ideal behavior in varied domains of life, as becomes evident through an analysis of the conceptualization of pain in Bariba thought. The subject of pain and the code of behavior surrounding painful experiences evokes from informants a cognitive map of honor and shame rather than a discussion of pain per se (cf. Sargent 1984). Thus, when interviewed regarding the reaction of Bariba hospital patients to surgical pain, a Bariba physician responded by quoting a Bariba proverb: *sekuru ka go go buram bo* [between death and shame, death has the greater beauty].

Asked to interpret this proverb, he explained that a Bariba who displays pain shows cowardice. Cowardice, in Bariba tradition, is the essence of shame (*sekuru*) and rather than live in shame, a true Bariba would kill himself.

Further pursuit of this line of thought demonstrated ubiquitous familiarity with the proverb and consistency in interpretation among both rural and urban informants. Examples given by informants to illustrate the meaning of the proverb were drawn from a set of categories of behavior described by informants in both settings:

1. The ideal behavior of the Bariba warrior; in this example, a scenario is described such as that where a Bariba chief leads his warriors

into battle. All are killed but he remains alive. Rather than return, having "eaten shame," he will kill himself with honor, thus preserving the respect of the community for his choice.

2. The ideal behavior of the thief; theft is uniformly offered as an example of shameful behavior among Bariba. To be revealed as a thief should be so shameful as to provoke suicide. Moreover, the person wrongfully accused of theft would theoretically commit suicide before the accusation became public. This example was provided in two forms—one a scenario in which a villager stole a neighbor's sheep. In this case the thief would face a public expose in which he would be paraded through the village carrying a sheep on his shoulders. According to informants, migration to another country or suicide would be the only means of living with such shame. In a second construction, an urban official was falsely accused of embezzlement and taken to the police headquarters twice for questioning. Rather than face such dishonor again, he would prefer to die.

3. The ideal behavior in cases of adultery; according to tradition, the man whose wife leaves him for another man should cut off his finger, and send it to his wife and her love. This finger indicates the commitment of the aggrieved spouse to protect his honor. If the wife returns home immediately, no further action may be taken. However, in the event that she does not return, the husband may kill the wife and lover with poisoned arrows, and then stab himself in the thigh with an arrow, thus provoking his own death.

4. The ideal behavior in cases of affliction; the woman in childbirth is expected to endure labor and delivery without any expression of discomfort. Ideally, she will not display to friends or relatives that she is in labor, will deliver alone, and will call for help only to cut the umbilical cord. A woman in labor who expresses pain is denigrated for she brings shame to the family of both the woman and her husband. For women, ideal behavior during childbirth is the key example offered of courageous behavior. For men, accidents and war wounds are cited as instances where a man may suffer excruciating pain. In such cases the ideal dictates indifference, lack of manifest response, and attempts to continue usual routine in spite of debility and pain.

Interestingly, discussions of affliction were always peripheral to the topic of courage in general. Unstructured interviewing which initially broached the subject of Bariba response to pain universally was diverted by informants to a commentary on Bariba courage—that of men in war and women in childbirth. Proverbs and general remarks on shame and honor ensued. Attempts to direct the informant back to the topic of pain led to an elaboration of that which is shameful in Bariba life, usually theft, adultery and incest. Inappropriate behavior in response to pain was added as a secondary category of shameful behavior, following upon the primary categories which involve ruptures of social relations.

Bariba who participated in discussions of the Bariba conception of the appropriate response to pain suggested that the Bariba capacity to remain impassive when in pain displays the superiority of the Bariba over their neighbors. When asked to contrast pain response by ethnic group, all Bariba interviewed commented disparagingly on the behavior of southerners (Fon, Yoruba); the shameful behavior of southern women during childbirth was a common example given of behavior unworthy of respect. Although rural women often have merely hearsay evidence regarding the behavior of other women at birth, urban women who had delivered at the hospital had personal observation as a basis for their conclusions, based on the proximity of women waiting in the corridors of the maternity clinic while in labor. Fon women themselves claimed that a marked verbal response to pain in childbirth is necessary in order to speed delivery and, further, to demonstrate to the father of the child the ordeal which the woman is suffering. Bariba midwives also criticized European women, who (they had heard) were fearful during labor and, moreover, allowed men to be present.

Clearly, the ideal pain response to Bariba is stoicism. But to what extent do Bariba women actually adhere to the ideal? Observation of over 50 deliveries in a rural community suggested that an overwhelming majority of women approached the ideal behavior during labor. Most women did not stop working at routine tasks until the onset of the second stage of labor, and only one woman openly complained of discomfort during delivery. This woman was criticized at length by her sisters, who claimed that after nine deliveries, she was still a coward and nothing could be done with her.

Examples of women who manifest remarkable courage during childbirth abound. While I was in the field, one Bariba woman bore twins, one of whom had died *in utero*. I transported her to a nearby urban clinic, where the dead twin was extracted by a nurse who used no anesthetic. The woman remained impassive throughout the procedure, provoking impressed comments from the non-Bariba staff, who commented that Bariba women are similarly stoical during manual extractions of the placenta. In general, hospital staff substantiated the Bariba perspective that Bariba rarely show or express pain and are loath to discuss the subject except insofar as discussion is necessary to describe a condition to a healer or hospital staff in order to request treatment. Two nurse-midwives at the Parakou hospital noted that Bariba women are remarkably stoical. One commented that after spending many years at maternity clinics in a Bariba region, she was transferred to the south of the country and was struck by the markedly different behavior of clinics from southern ethnic groups, who expressed pain vociferously. This midwife suggested that in her observation, southern women who live in the north express their admiration of northern women in the clinics and try to adopt the demeanor of these women during labor.

It is instructive to examine those features of the socialization process which may explain the manner in which pain is characteristically expressed in Bariba society. Informants were interviewed regarding the method by which Bariba learn to suppress a verbal or behavioral response to pain. Male informants responded consistently that circumcision provided the primary opportunity for boys to learn the appropriate behavior during a painful experience, while women cited clitoridectomy as the critical incident in their lives which formed their response to pain. One informant, Lafia Roger, a man now in his late fifties and a high-ranking official in Parakou, explained the process as follows:

> The Bariba realize that life consists of many ordeals. The tests of life for a man are war, the burden of his friends and relatives, and protecting the honor of his family. The tests of life for a woman are excision, defloration, birth, and protecting her children. Initiation prepares boys and girls to endure the tests ahead.

Formerly, boys aged 9 to 11 were circumcised in groups. Lafia recalled his own initiation, describing how the initiate had been advised long before the event, that he is expected to remain impassive throughout the circumcision, that if he grimaces, cries, or jerks during the procedure, he will bring unending shame to his family. During the ceremony, the initiate sits on a rock. His father's brother or mother's brother (the latter being the most intimidating) stands before the boy, staring into his eyes, compelling him not to blink or cry. As the circumciser proceeds, the family's praise singer sings the praises of the courageous boy and his family. To Lafia, this event epitomizes the merging of pain, courage, and honor.

Clitoridectomy, practiced on girls prior to puberty, represents a similar procedure for women, although the girls are not sanctioned for crying (see Sargent 1982:35 for details of clitoridectomy). Currently, clitoridectomy is illegal, although the practice continues, primarily in rural areas. Women in their twenties and thirties who reflected on their experience with clitoridectomy commented that they were encouraged to be brave and praised for not crying.

Kora Zaliatou, born and raised in Parakou but now living in a village, remarked that nothing in life is as excruciatingly painful as clitoridectomy. After circumcision, she said, no pain will overwhelm a person. A similar attitude was expressed by many women questioned regarding their feelings during such potentially painful experiences as delivery who noted that they felt significant pain, but that a woman feeling pain would "master herself," and not allow the pain to take control of her body.

Although the emphasis on stoicism seems to be somewhat greater for men than women (women are believed to be generally more emotional and less controlled than men), both sexes are expected to attempt the ideal, and are provided with both verbal instructions and role models for doing so. Circumcision initiates, as described previously, are told in detail the nature of the procedure to which they will be subjected, the feelings they will experience, the response which they are expected to manifest. Although not all children have observed initiations prior to their own, they have had ample opportunity to observe adults and older children reacting to other types of pain-provoking experiences. Moreover, they have been exposed to mockeries of those who complain and praises of those who perform with courage, and have received corresponding admonitions or praises when hurt or sick themselves. Thus, as one Bariba trader in town recalled, if a child has a thorn stuck in his hand and begins to cry, he will be told not to fuss or "you'll never be king." Another informant noted that as one grows up, a sort of auto-suggestion occurs in view of pain. One remembers the mockery attendant upon complaint and the urge to express the feeling dissipates, given that "people don't say anything if you behave correctly but if you cry, since they have nothing else to do in a village, they will talk about that."

Similarly, girls observe as they grow up that the pregnant women in the household do not indicate that they are in labor, that one never hears any expressions of pain while the women are delivering, and that women are praised subsequent to delivery for such behavior. Men recount admiring tales of their wives, who managed to deliver without the husband even knowing that they were in labor until the newborn began to cry. In addition, a woman who is pregnant for the first time is thoroughly instructed by more experienced female friends and relatives regarding the feelings that she will experience during labor and the appropriate behavior during delivery. Thus she will be told that she must continue her routine tasks about the house until she can no longer stand up, at which time she should go alone to a room of the house; when she feels the urge to push, she should kneel until she delivers. At that time, someone will come to assist her. This combination of instruction and example, according to Bariba women of reproductive age interviewed in the rural area of Pehunko, suffices to enable a woman to manage her delivery without expressing fears and discomfort.

Birth in the Hospital Setting

As initiation rituals decline in prevalence, one might expect a parallel relinquishing of emphasis on stoicism or "absence of manifest behavior" in response to pain. To date, this is not evident, either in home or hospital deliveries. Women in Parakou who were asked to compare home and hospital birth settings observed that labor and delivery, in whatever context, require courage in the face of pain. Hospital delivery thus far is not seen as either more or less painful than home delivery, nor do women perceive that stoicism is less requisite at a hospital birth. However, features of the hospital setting are often cited as especially distressing. These features include the lack of privacy for the woman in labor, the presence of male staff, the restrictions on companionship in the delivery room, and the authoritative attitude of personnel. Although women uniformly expressed the view that the hospital will save you if you suffer and that hospital delivery is safer for mother and child, pain relief did not emerge as a facet of the diminished suffering experienced at the hospital. Rather, women remarked that pain is an intrinsic aspect of birth and must be "managed" by the woman in labor. Two women remarked specifically that a woman delivering at the hospital suffered intense shame, in addition to pain, because of her exposed genitals; however, several others contradicted this view, stating that shame is irrelevant on the day of delivery and that a woman in labor cannot close her thighs to anyone, even a male physician.

In assessing the implications of hospital delivery for the pain response among women in labor, Romalis offers a pessimistic view suggesting that

The kinds of social and psychological supports that women are given in primitive and peasant societies . . . unquestionably aid the management of pain without medication. When the support systems in traditional societies are eroded, there is increasing reliance on pharmacological and surgical management. In Northern Thailand, for example, the woman has traditionally been accompanied in labor by her parents, children, and husband, who have played a vital role by providing physical and psychological support. With modernization, the wealthier middle- and upper-class families are now opting for "safer" hospitals/births which exclude the family (Muecke 1976). This trend parallels that of many countries in the developing world and surely has profound implications for a woman. Whereas life crises, like death and birth, were always handled by the family within the home, they are now becoming the responsibility of impersonal institutions (1981:12).

Similarly, Rothman argues that hospital delivery seems to be experienced as more painful than home delivery due to such factors as lack of emotional support, absence of distraction and confinement to bed (Rothman 1981:162).

The Bariba women who deliver in Parakou currently do not seem to experience a hospital delivery as more painful than a home birth. However, a key factor in this issue may relate to the practicality of reliance on pharmacological and surgical management of birth mentioned by Romalis and Rothman. To date, the Parakou hospitals and clinics are inadequately stocked and understaffed. Supply of medications and equipment is notoriously undependable and analgesics are rarely approved for maternity patients. Certainly there is not yet any routine use of analgesics for women in labor. There is an increasing awareness among the urban population that such medications exist, due to the lively advertising campaign for aspirin and related products; however, these drugs seem to be conceptualized as fever-reducers and remedies for headache rather than as gynecological or obstetrical therapies.

Zborowski has described two differing attitudes towards various types of pain. He states that these may be categorized as pain expectancy and pain avoidance:

> Pain expectancy is anticipation of pain as being avoidable in a given situation, for instance, in childbirth, in sports activities or in battle. Pain acceptance is characterized by a willingness to experience pain. This attitude is manifested mostly as an inevitable component of culturally accepted experiences, for instance, as part of initiation rites or part of medical treatment. . . . Labor pain is expected as part of childbirth, but while in one culture, such as in the United States, it is not accepted and therefore various means are used to alleviate it, in some other cultures, for instance in Poland, it is not only expected but also accepted, and consequently nothing or little is done to relieve it (1978:281).

Given the lack of available analgesics and general limitations of the hospital service, Bariba women who deliver at the Parakou hospital continue to hold the customary perspective that pain at birth is unavoidable and cannot be altered by outside intervention. Pain control therefore remains the province of the woman herself.

Conclusion

Reproduction, for Bariba women, involves a display of women's power, represented through the medium of birth seen as heroic exploit. Women find in childbirth the opportunity to demonstrate both honor and courage, highly valued virtues in Bariba society. Men, by contrast, have opportunities to demonstrate these qualities in the domains of hunting and warfare. It appears that for both men and women, initiation rites (circumcision and clitoridectomy respectively) provide initial training for management and response to pain. It is not yet clear whether the decline in initiations in response to government prohibitions will alter the expected behavior for those confronted with other painful ordeals.

Although the theme of honor and courage remains evident among women who deliver at urban hospitals, it appears attenuated in relation to other concerns, referred to above among the Agendas informing medical choices. While rural women explain that they prefer not to deliver in clinics for reasons involving honor, shame, and cosmological concerns, and glorify the woman who delivers alone with no sign of pain or fear of danger, urban women offer a variety of reasons to justify their decision to deliver in the hospital. These include greater competence of hospital personnel, safety, prestige, and associated desires to avoid "peasant" behaviors such as home birth. Government influence emerges in this paradigm shift, as government efforts to encourage hospital delivery and to invest government institutions with control over birth have contributed to public perceptions of the relative merits in home and hospital delivery.

Public health policy supports the elimination of home delivery and the diminishing of household responsibility for reproduction. Currently, although the structural limitations of the government hospital constrain professional dominance of birth, the ideology of medical management of obstetrics by specialists is certainly manifest among nurse-midwives and physicians, who are trained according to the premises of cosmopolitan medicine. Technological intervention at birth is likely to increase as infrastructural constraints are reduced. Such intervention is likely to be accompanied (as Rothman notes) by an even greater limitation of family participation at delivery, bed confinement for the woman in labor, and increased reliance on pharmacological management at birth. In turn, one would expect to find that the sense of control that Bariba women now express when they discuss their birth experiences will diminish. This decreased control (both structural and perceived) may well contribute to a reinterpretation of the meaning of pain and to a reformulation of expected behavior for Bariba women at delivery.

References Cited

Janzen, John. 1987. Therapy Management: Concept, Reality, Process. Medical Anthropology Quarterly (New Series) 1(1):68–84.

Feierman, Steven. 1985. Struggles for Control: The Social Roots of Health and Healing in Modern Africa. African Studies Review 28(2–3):73–149.

Sargent, Carolyn. 1982. The Cultural Context of Therapeutic Choice. Obstetrical Care Decisions Among the Bariba of Benin. Dordrecht, Holland: D. Reidel Publishing Co.

_____. 1984. Between Death and Shame. Dimensions of Pain in Bariba Culture. Special Issue, Social Science and Medicine 19(12):1299-1304.

5

The Politics of Children: Fosterage and the Social Management of Fertility Among the Mende of Sierra Leone

Caroline Bledsoe

Sub-Saharan African fertility rates remain high, despite forces of modernization and urbanization which might be expected to decrease the utility of children as subsistence laborers and increase their costs of maintenance and education. However, many explanations of high African fertility make two incorrect assumptions. First, they assume that prenatal methods of control are the primary means used to regulate family size and composition. A notable effort to deal with post-natal methods is that of Scrimshaw (1978), who treats infanticide as a way for economically-pressed couples lacking adequate forms of birth control to reduce their completed family size (see also Scheper-Hughes 1987). This essay examines child fosterage, another post-natal method of managing family size and composition. Unlike infanticide, fosterage—one of the most striking features of African families—is not an extreme, irreversable adjustment; it can be done and undone a number of times, even with the same child, to meet new exigencies.

The second erroneous assumption most fertility theories make is that families that biologically bear children must also bear the economic consequences of raising them. This makes parents the focus of reproduction: why they want children, how they pay costs, and when they derive benefits. Conversely, the children whom parents bear biologically are treated as the only ones from whom they can later draw support.[1]

Widespread West African fosterage—sending children away from their natal homes to be raised or educated—challenges these assumptions. In fact, support for, and benefits from, raising children are rarely confined exclusively to parents. Among the Mende of Sierra Leone, who have high rates of fosterage even for African groups, many people have responsibility toward, and can demand benefits from, children.

Yet the relationship of fosterage (or other forms of investing in children) to fertility is not straightforward. We must spell out the social complexities of post-natal methods of family size control if we are to understand their relationship to fertility patterns. To this end, the chapter moves beyond the more mechanical aspects of child-caretaker relations. It shows that although fosterage is one way to gain benefits from children, neither a foster child nor, for that matter, a natural child yield guaranteed benefits to caretakers. Instead, adults have a much more dynamic yet problematic view of children: as potential sources of support, not infallible ones. People must try to activate rights and obligations to secure benefits. Expanding reproduction to include the regulation and management of family size and composition through a variety of post-natal means reveals reproduction less as an event than a process: one oriented less toward the past than the future. I show how adults, seeking to alleviate risk and future uncertainty, try to stake claims in children, especially those with promise for success in later life.

In terms of more general implications, I stress the importance of sociopolitical processes of negotiating benefits from children. Mende adults and children can tinker with their relationships, creating new ties, strengthening old ones, and redefining burdensome ones. Thus, cultural labels such as kinship and fosterage are best viewed not as relationships that compel future support, but as idioms for making demands or asserting claims with respect to children.

Background

According to an analysis of the 1974 census (Thomas 1983), the Mende number 799,905: 30 percent of the country's population. Many Mende still practice slash-and-burn rice agriculture, though income from trading, cash cropping, and diamond mining have intensified the purchase of imported staples. Prestige generally accrues from living in new houses in large towns and from access to modern consumer goods such as imported foods. Marriage may be polygynous, especially in wealthy or chiefly families, and family descent is ideally patrilineal, although practice often differs. Technically a father is responsible for his children's cash costs, but his wives pay many of their children's expenses out of their own incomes from trading or wage work.

Data for the chapter come from a 1981–82 ethnographic study in a semi-urban Mende town of about 4,400 in the Eastern Province of Sierra Leone, and from a return trip in 1985 to a larger town in the Southern Province. Qualitative methods consisted of open-ended interviews, participant observation, case studies, collecting family genealogies and diaries, and so on. There were two primary sources of quantitative data. A 1982 survey contained information on all the children (present, away, and dead) born to 165 women aged 18 to 49 in the survey households, and on children for whom they were caring. A 1985 survey was conducted in a larger town of about 35,000. It was based on interviews with about 852 women aged 15 to 60 in selected households.

The town studied in 1981–82 is the main one from which present material is drawn. Its population was about 80 percent Muslim and 15 percent Christian. It had a daily market and several primary schools supported by Christian and Muslim missions and by the government. It also has a secondary school. Local children enrolled in these schools, but many were fostered out elsewhere for schooling. Similarly, many from outlying rural areas had come to live with guardians to attend school or to take up apprenticeships with local carpenters, masoners, drivers, and tailors.

The specific area studied, of course, is part of a wider sociopolitical context. Since precolonial times, status and wealth in Africa have stemmed generally from the control of people rather than land (see also J. Goody 1971, Kopytoff and Miers 1977, Bledsoe 1980b). Rank rested on a patrons' ability to attract dependent clients and wives who produced economic surpluses to attract other dependents who, in turn, produced more surpluses.[2] Individuals attempted to gain status not by escaping the patronage hierarchy and attaining a dangerous state of "independence," but by ascending within it: acquiring higher status patrons as well as dependents of their own. In other words, patrons needed patrons and clients needed clients.

Under the British colonial regime, local polities in Sierra Leone were incorporated into a system of chieftaincies within the national Parliamentary and Presidential system. But the national structure, despite its formal nomenclature, has remained basically a patron-client system. Jobs, scholarships, and other valued resources trickle down through personal ties to powerful brokers who can intervene with national institutions (see Murphy 1981 and Handwerker 1987 for Liberian cases). While this modern system offers enticing opportunities for wealth and advancement, court cases that strip people of land, property, and dependents are commonly trumped up against those known to have weakly developed patronage support. Rural people in particular are vulnerable. They need powerful intermediaries to provide them with outside resources gained from high position, yet buffer them from heavy-handed government officials who demand excessive taxes from them and pressure them for "contributions" to building projects that benefit the administrative elite.

Therefore, low status people must take on patrons as protection against other patrons to whom they are not attached.

With precipitous declines in the national economy, people have even greater need for patrons well connected to the urban and government bureaucracies to bypass cumbersome bureaucratic channels during shortages of food, money, and petrol. They also have greater need for patrons in the international world: for travel, jobs, and access to hard foreign currency.

Fosterage

Mende adults want children for labor and future support. But within this political climate of uncertainty, instability, and patronage, children are also valued for their links to powerful patrons and other families. Apparently the Mende had a concept of "development" (*tEE-guloma*) before they were incorporated into the colony of Sierra Leone. It referred to growing bigger farms and accreting more family members. They still use the term today, but have given it new meaning. They now hope that young people will "develop" the family's social standing and access to resources through formal schooling.

Today, most young people yearn to be "civilized" (*pu*—'modern,' 'civilized'): to live not in rural villages, but in "open places" where knowledge of the outside world is said to uplift society. They want to be literate; wear well-tailored Western-style clothes; speak English and Krio, the national lingua francas; and acquire civil service or business jobs where they earn regular monthly wages, instead of relying on irregular seasonal harvests.

Parents try to "develop" promising children so they can participate in the "civilized" world, and bring back benefits from it. Fosterage is a pivotal strategy whereby people attempt to "develop" promising future patrons. Parents try to send their children to more "civilized" guardians who can pull up fostered children to their own level. In the ideal, if such a child indeed succeeds in this environment, the guardians, seeing his yet greater potential, may send him up to their own high status patrons, and so on. While guardians try eventually to claim some of the child's "benefits," the parents' ultimate rewards from this "developed" child are deemed much greater than if they had not fostered out the child.

Like wives, foster children also provide political links between groups. Even for women, the legal minors of husbands and fathers, the ability to arrange advantageous fosterage situations for their own children or to foster in children, can bolster their positions within the household and the community (see also Etienne 1983; Bledsoe, MS). In contrast to the firmly held belief in Western society that children need stable parental figures throughout their childhood, most Mende would argue the opposite: the truly unfortunate children are those who have not been sent away from home to advance.

Mende children are seldom "adopted" in the legal sense. They can be brought back to parents when needed or even sent out to other guardians for different purposes. For simplicity, my household survey defined as fosters those children living in households apart from their biological mothers. (See Page's effort [in press] to develop a more fine-grained typology). Yet the term "fosterage" is difficult to apply concisely to the Mende context. My definition, for example, would not classify as fosters those children living in the same household with their mothers, but cared for by subfertile co-wives. On the other hand, children I classify as fosters are not seen as such in the cultural context. A woman raising her sister's child will likely insist that this is her "own" child, an appellation consistent with African classificatory kinship. And despite the patrilineal ideology, I classify as fosters those children living with their fathers but not their own mothers because of the likelihood of differential treatment; their fathers' other wives may demand more work from them, and allow them fewer resources, than their own children.

The Mende distinguish between two principal kinds of fosterage. The first involves sending out small children simply to be "raised" (*a ngi gbuang*—'he/she raises him/her up') or "minded": what E. Goody (1982) calls "nurturant" fosterage (see also Bledsoe and Isiugo-Abanihe, in press), until they reach what the Mende regard as an educable age, about 5 to 7. The second, for older children, involves training or learning for life (*kaa*): learning Arabic (Bledsoe and Robey 1986) or a trade (both most common for boys) or attending Western schools. For schooling or trade apprenticeships, children are commonly sent to relatives, friends, or patrons in large towns where good schools and skilled urban tradesmen are located. Girls are commonly sent for training in cooking, housekeeping, and childcare. Increasingly they are sent for schooling, though their dropout rates are much higher than those of boys. Just as the best opportunities for training boys now lie in urban areas, parents also try to send their daughters to urban areas to learn to keep a modern house.

Census as well as survey data reveal that fosterage is common in Mende areas (see also Isaac and Conrad 1982). Of all the children under 18 living in the households I surveyed in 1982, 39 percent were without their mothers, while 34 percent of the living children born to women in the survey were currently away. Many leave quite young. Of the living children under five born to women in the survey, 22.5 percent were currently away. Of these, one fourth had left before the age of two, and nearly half before three. However, these figures are low, compared to other Mende areas: 1974 national census figures revealed that in some southern chiefdoms, over 50 percent of the children of women between 15 and 19—mostly children under two—were away from their biological mothers. (The number of weanlings away appears high, even compared to other African societies. See Page [in press] for some comparative figures.)

The likelihood of being fostered out increases with the child's age. In my survey, 27.8 percent from ages 6 to 10 were away, as were 45.9 percent of the children from 11 to 15. My data suggest that children are being sent out at increasingly younger ages. However, fosterage is so common, including sending a young child to the grandmother or aunt after weaning or a divorce, that the younger women may better remember fosterage events because they occurred more recently.

The most salient caretakers of young children are "grannies." A "granny" can be any older woman, regardless of her exact relationship to the child, although it is frequently the mother's mother. A granny who takes in a small child hopes for financial support from the child's parents. She also hopes for support from the child himself as he matures and as she becomes feeble.

Because the Mende maintain that a child cannot learn much before the "age of sense," around age six, they are willing to send younger children out to rural grannies who have little status or access to schools. When children are ready for schooling or other training, however, being with a granny is considered disadvantageous, because grannies are said to spoil children who need, at this age, to buckle down to learn. Parents usually try to bring them back or send them on to younger, more urban caretakers. These social needs are reflected quantitatively. In my survey, almost half (48 percent) of the fosters ages 0 to 5 were with grannies, compared to only 21 percent of fostered children 6 and over; the latter were overwhelmingly children whose parents were not married—that is, parents who were hard-pressed to care for their children, or who wanted to remove from their new spouses' views the awkward reminders of their previous unions.

The Implications of Fosterage
for Costs and Benefits of Children

Parents' Perspectives

The fact that reproduction can be regulated socially through fosterage minimizes the costs of raising children, making them to a large extent independent of parents' biological fertility (see also Caldwell 1977; Okore

1977; Sembajwe 1977; Fapohunda 1978; Oppong and Bleek 1982; and Page MS). A Mende man stated this lucidly:

> One does not necessarily bear the burden of raising one's children. They are sent out so parents don't face the problem of educating them or providing for them or suffer any problem emanating from their large family size. On the contrary, they [the parents] gain.

Another man drew attention to the utility of fostering out children during difficult times such as seasonal hardships or when several children are born in rapid succession:

> All this [fosterage] is to relieve the boarding and care expenses, because if the parents have a child with them and a young baby, they will have difficulty in taking care of both children. So what they do is to find somebody to take care of the older one while they live with the younger one. They are trying to release the boarding expenses, care, lodging, all these things. But as long as the child is staying with another person, that person undergoes the expenses. Parents don't pay anything. Nothing at all. [Note: This is not always the case.]

Reducing child raising costs helps sustain a high demand for children, making childbearers less interested in learning about or using birth control. Quantitative support for this is found in logistic regression analyses of the two large household surveys conducted in 1982 and 1985. For women, one of the features most closely associated with whether they were currently fostering out any children was high fertility ($p = .04$ in the 1985 survey). Conversely, one of the features most closely associated with fostering in children was low fertility ($p = .03$).[3]

Precise causal links for these associations, however, are hard to identify. Indeed, potential guardians such as grannies who hope to benefit from other children may support or even demand high fertility from childbearers. Parents recognize, moreover, that unforseen situations will arise inevitably: they may divorce; a sibling may die, leaving several children; a friend may prove barren or may experience child loss; the farm may be unproductive one year; the local primary school may close; and so on. All these may necessitate fosterage.

To complicate the interaction, fosterage and fertility may affect each other concurrently (see Isiugo-Abanihe 1985): parents who send away children because of high fertility can afford to bear more. When I asked one man whether people send their children away because of economic problems—or if they feel free to have children because they know fosterage is possible—he replied:

If you have a sister, a brother, or an uncle, you can send any of your children to them, and they cannot refuse them. So you know ahead of time, even when you have one or two children at first, that if you have 5 or 6 more, you can send them out. We are not worried about taking care of them [children]. We just know that every child can be raised in a home, whether [with] the born family or the relatives. That's why we have the extended family. We are interested in having children. It is very good to see them. They are children, and I will not try to stop giving birth to them. Everybody knows that they will give birth to children, and if they are not capable of bringing them up, they can give them out to relatives to be taken care of. We know that. If you are reproducing while your elder sister is without children, you can distribute them to keep the family ties firm.

Because fosterage is so acceptable culturally, posing a definitive causal relationship between fosterage and fertility becomes a sterile exercise. Indeed, to the Mende, the two are inextricably linked aspects of social reproduction.

This assertion finds further support in questions of the "quality" of children. Fosterage is not simply a distressful measure of last resort wherein parents react to the economic hardships of high fertility; it can have highly positive incentives (see also Frank 1984, Isiugo-Abanihe 1985). Indeed, parents consider fertility useless unless the child is enhanced through social means. Fosterage can give children training they could not otherwise obtain and, through their social mobility, broaden a family's sources of potential future support. (E. Goody 1982 and Oppong 1973, among others, also show that educational advantages may accrue to fostered children.) Parents hope that the education and contacts gained from fosterage will help some of their children to become prominent businessmen or civil servants and to contract advantageous marriages. These children can then help the rest of the family to progress in the modern world and to forestall trouble with government authorities or tax collectors. Parents also try to create diversity in the training and contacts their various children. A man explained:

It is important to have many children. First, to help the younger ones, and secondly, to help you at your old age, so when you are old, you will have support coming from different angles or sources. Let's say your first son sent you a bag of rice, you have a daughter who is a nurse [to] provide medicine, another child is a Permanent Secretary who will send money for you to maintain the house, and so on.

Parents also hope to improve their relationships with individuals to whom they send children, particularly individuals of prestige and position.

Many try to give children to patrons to betoken their dependence. In fact, some of the most salient reasons for fostering children involve adults' attempts to establish or strengthen advantageous relationships with other adults, rather than to derive direct utility from the children themselves. For example, in Liberia indigenous children were sent to the capital city to be educated and incorporated into the national system dominated by Americo-Liberians. These children became mediators for their rural people with the Americo-Liberians, whom villagers regarded as hostile, punitive elites (Murphy 1981). In the end, fosterage, like fertility, allows parents to build up a base of personal power vis-a-vis spouses, in-laws, and even rivalrous kin, and to build a wide regional network of ties that can yield significant benefits from the modern sector. Such strong positive incentives help explain why even people with only a few children often foster them out.

Fosterage strategies of mobility for older children produce important lines of social and geographic stratification. At each upward step, the children's lower status marked them as domestic servants for more educated or urban families. This in turn means that the greater the status differential between the sending and receiving families, the less the foster children will be treated like the guardian's own children, and the more hardship they are likely to undergo. The tradeoff is the possibility of an incremental rise in the child's adult status. Similar patterns arose historically in Europe, despite the different contexts. As McCracken explains for Tudor England:

> Each rank, even noble ones, could hope that the experience gained in a home superior to their own would give the child a sophistication, breadth of outlook, and opportunity for advancement that they themselves could not provide (p. 311).

The intriguing aspect of these social and geographic mobility strategies is that throughout the entire social hierarchy, parents try to send their own older children to more urban areas with people of higher social and educational status, while simultaneously taking in children from more rural areas (or from households of lesser status), whose parents also seek more "modern" opportunities for them. There is clear numerical support for this. My 1982 survey asked guardians about the status ("living conditions") of their household versus that from which foster children had come and parents about the status of their household versus that where they had sent their out-fostered children. Taking all 176 in-fostered and out-fostered children under 16 years of age, 51 percent were in better situations than previously, compared to only 17 percent in worse conditions. (Thirty-two percent were in households of the same status.)

Guardians' Perspectives

Just as parents can shift the burdens of child care to better-placed guardians, guardians have much to gain from foster children. Such children perform household and marketing chores, take care of smaller children, and so on. Besides these short-term gains, guardians can try to make future claims on their former fostered children's monetary and political assistance, much as parents can.

At some point in their lives, practically all adults foster in some children who are not their own, often because of kinship ties, but also through ties of friendship or patronage. This gives them leverage for future support unobtainable solely through biological chance—their own fertility, their children's possible mortality, the age and sex of their surviving children, etc. They also gain social insurance against the possibility that their own children will not support them. In the Mende view, the position of a person who has not invested in other people's children is almost as precarious as that of a person who has remained childless. (Findley and Diallo 1988 argue cogently that Malinke guardians actually try to dilute the children's ties with their parents.)

Fosterage per se is only one way to invest in other people's children. Women can pay school fees for children known to be clever in school or invite them to eat when they are hungry, using these actions as a basis for future requests for assistance. Typically, people who made any contribution at all to a young wage earner's upbringing—school fees, food, even a bowl of rice one day—will come to him for assistance because of their help (or claimed help) during his formative years. Although many students face enormous economic difficulties, the brightest ones can collect what they claim as "school expenses" many times over, spending excess money on clothes, cigarettes, and "amplifier dances," featuring Highlife music blared through enormous speakers. Yet many adults tolerate this embezzlement. What the children actually do with the money matters less to them than the fact that their contributions establish a basis for making claims on potentially powerful individuals. In effect, both parents and guardians are choosing to invest in children, depending on the children's demonstrated potentials, and their own circumstances, after the initial fertility act.

Of course, like parents, guardians incur costs. Small children sometimes require expensive medical treatment and make heavy demands on female labor. But by virtue of their positions in the household, older foster children cost their guardians less than "born" children of women in the household. Since older fosters tend to come from households of lower status than those of the guardians, they are assigned the most time consuming and burdensome chores (see also Schildkrout 1973 and Etienne 1983), and they tend to be engaged in "training" for household skills (girls) or trade apprenticeships (boys), in which they provide labor for their masters. The costs of fosters are also offset in the long term by potential reciprocity. Even older "grannies" who take in small children expect reciprocity: from the children's parents in the present and from the children themselves in the future, should the "grannies" survive to "feeble old age." In contrast, foster children brought in to attend school are more expensive in the short term to guardians than children engaged in "home training." But the costs of fostering them are mitigated by the possibility of greater future rewards.

Moreover, fosters cost less to raise than "born" children because, on the whole, they receive fewer household resources. If sent to school by guardians, they usually attend less prestigious (i.e., less expensive) schools. When they get sick, their complaints may be dismissed as faking to avoid work; in contrast, mothers take their own children's complaints more seriously. Foster children also receive less food, especially protein, from the household than "born" children. Although it is common for all the children within a certain age group to eat together out of a large basin, mothers usually see that their own children get the choicest bits of food. And snacks, comprising a large proportion of children's diets, are given more to the "born" children, whether through intention or simple oversight. Many older foster children forage largely for themselves by stealing, overcharging marketing customers, eating with friends, and so on (Bledsoe 1983, Bledsoe et al. MS).

It is also quite easy with any children, but perhaps especially with fosters, to scale down expenditures to meet current exigencies. As one man explained, the tightening economic situation means that he cannot take in outside children so much any more. Instead, he reduces his investments, both in terms of whom he helps, as well as the amount he gives. When I talked to him, he was fostering no outside children, but he was helping his sister with some of her children's school expenses.

Fostering Out and In Simultaneously

I have made the case that by fostering out their children, parents lose their own children's labor; but they can generally replace it with labor of children from "less developed" homes. Moreover, fosterage also has clear positive incentives for the children's "development." Parents usually lack the resources to "develop" their children further than their own socioeconomic level. Consequently, it is to the child's—and the parent's—advantage to arrange a fosterage with more "developed" guardians who can pull the child up to their own level. While this gives the guardians a claim to a share of the child's resources in the future, the net returns to the parents from this child are much greater.

Because both biological parents and guardians can try to claim benefits from successful children in the future, parents commonly foster in children while simultaneously fostering out some of their own to other people. Fostering in an older child, especially a girl, may actually support a woman's own high fertility. A fostered girl can take care of her guardian's young children, while releasing her to pursue money-making enterprises: thus, allowing her to send her own children away to school in larger towns. In effect, then, parents may foster in children in order to send away their own.

This suggests that parents can manage without their children's labor because they can usually replace it with that of foster children from areas yet more rural areas than their own: children whose parents also seek more "modern" opportunities for them. (Isaac and Conrad 1982, however, suggest that there is a finite supply of children: as we might predict, they found a lower ratio of foster children to "born" children in rural areas than in the more urban area.) In the long term, however, parents are willing to give up short term labor for the possibility of future rewards and security from a child who went away to a better school than the one in their own town.

Finally, from the guardian's perspective, foster children, particularly older ones, are cheap to maintain, compared to their own children, as the above discussion has demonstrated. When combined, fosterage and fertility lessen the costs of reproduction.

How adults benefit from particular children depends on their own sex and life cycle characteristics as well as those of the children. Child receivers may be sub-fertile or need more children of a certain age or sex. Parents, on the other hand, tend to send certain kinds of children for fosterage when their own life situations demand it. They can also retrieve fostered-out children when they need them, or make demands on the children's earnings and labor when their benefits begin to exceed their liabilities. Often these strategies of sending and receiving children are closely interwoven. For example, a young mother who wishes to continue having children but finds it taxing can send her young children to her mother or foster in an older girl to help with child care. As she matures, she can demand that the household support several foster children to help her establish a small business or even bring back some of her older children to help. In her old age, she may foster in a young child, usually a girl, who helps her with household chores; and she can make demands on the child's parents for food, money, and medical care because she is fostering the child.

Fosterage Chains

Although the costs of children can be offset immediately by sending them away and perhaps taking in others that are cheaper to raise, one of the most interesting ways in which fosterage helps to sustain high fertility is that older children often assume the expenses of younger ones by taking them to raise. That is, parents can obligate certain children (their own or fosters) to repay favors by raising the parents' subsequent children.

Concerning sibling fosterage, grown independent children often take in their younger siblings and pay their school expenses. Here the ethic seems to be, "Your parents gave birth to you and made you what you are, so you, in turn, must take the burden of educating your siblings from them." The notion of "child spacing," which the Mende attribute to Western family planning advocates, is widely hailed as a means of reducing the costs of raising and educating children. It is hailed, however, not as a means of spreading out one's own costs over a longer time, but as a means of more easily shifting the responsibility of raising the younger children onto the older ones. Said one man who regretted that his own children were closely spaced:

> Say if my first child has started school since 1979, then I am expecting to send the other one in 1985. Then I would expect that the five or six years [spacing] would help me because by the time the other one finishes the secondary school, the other one might be starting, and I expect the moment you complete your secondary school, you would engage in some other work to earn you money. So that would help assist the younger one. [It would] enable the first born to help in educating the others.

A number of what I call "minding [fosterage] chains" occurred also when children who had been sent out to attend school were asked later to take in younger children of their guardians. These now-grown children were typically successful wage earners living in more urban locations than those of their former guardians (see also Caldwell 1977). One young man described his own case, wherein he was raising two older boys:

> Whatever I do for them, whether I pay their medical bills, whether I pay their school fees, all these things, nobody is going to help me. So that means that their parents are released from their expenses. I am taking that up. It is an obligation. Because I was taken care of by my other

relatives they sent me to my uncle. The last boy I have in the house is
my uncle's son. He is dead now, so they said, "OK, your uncle took care
of you, so you take care of that one [his son]."

Such strategies also provide a form of insurance, in the event that
the parent dies leaving young children. More importantly, they clearly
reflect strategies of social mobility in a hierarchical system based on
advancement through ties of dependency. In the ideal of family development, each generation can theoretically boost the family up to the
level of its most successful members. A guardian who helps a minded
child to move up in the world hopes that this child, in turn, will raise
the guardian's own children past his own new vantage point. Using
each new level as its "anchor" (as one young man put it, using an
English metaphor), the family "develops" by sending out new children
to ever-more advanced levels.

Regional Significance of Fosterage

Fosterage has important economic and social effects that extend well
beyond the household level. The net migration of younger children is
to more rural areas (where "grannies" tend to live); when children reach
six or so, there is a reverse migration, as they return to where their
parents live, or go to even more urban areas for training (Bledsoe and
Isiugo-Abanihe, in press).

These facts are significant beyond concerns with individual reproductive
couples. They reveal important regional relationships (rural vs. urban
or subsistence vs. cash economies) through which costs of child rearing
are spread. Small children tend to go toward more rural areas, until
they reach the age when they can be sent to school or apprenticed. At
that point, they move toward more urban areas. These shifts transfer
the primary costs of raising young children to the subsistence sector
and the costs of raising older children to urban areas. On the other
hand, grown children can remit modern urban benefits such as cash,
purchased goods, and legal assistance to rural parents or grandparents,
a fact of growing importance in an environment wherein older children's
utility as farm laborers is decreasing (Bledsoe and Isiugo-Abanihe in
press).

Toward the Social Construction
of Demographic Reality

The material presented suggests that the Mende do not need to make
fertility decisions early in their conjugal lives, basing their decisions on

estimates of how much each child will cost or yield. Fosterage provides a social means of compensating for biological limitations in response to present conditions and to anticipated future ones. It gives adults enormous flexibility in distributing the costs and benefits of children. Even people who are themselves parents readily foster in or assist other people's children to establish claims in a wide range of children. Fosterage is thus one manifestation of a much wider process of socially constructing a family after the fact of actual fertility. It allows adults to adjust continuously as family and household events unfold.

I have shown that high fertility is associated statistically with high fosterage rates within the specific Mende populations studied. However, the two are not linked directly on a more macro-level. Otherwise, the Mende, who have very high rates of fosterage, should have rates of fertility that are among the highest in Africa. Completed family size for the Mende (in both my surveys, women from 40 to 60 had borne about 5.7 children) is certainly not as large as in parts of East Africa, wherein fosterage rates are low (see Page, in press). Instead, fosterage must be treated as part of a more general issue: the management of family size and composition through social means.

The social management of reproduction rests on a crucial fact: although adults try to derive future benefits from children, they cannot rely on such support. Whereas we might expect a foster child to reciprocate later to a guardian (e.g., E. Goody 1982), in reality this guardian becomes one of many claimants, all of whom it is impossible to satisfy. Highly successful urbanites learn quickly to make short, unannounced visits to their rural homes to avoid long lines of people who claim to have been instrumental to their success. Yet even biological parenthood does not guarantee support (see also Cain 1982). There are some obvious risks: children may not achieve the educational or employment goals their parents expect of them and some children will die before reaching adulthood. But potential benefits from the children will be diverted in more subtle ways as well. Relatives or friends will likely ask for children— requests that parents cannot gracefully deny. And children themselves will try to avoid their parents' claims in ongoing efforts to balance the demands of their natal and conjugal families.

Some of these failures to meet kinship or fosterage obligations un- doubtedly stem from national economic problems of recession and inflation, which decrease the resources of young wage earners. But simply achieving success in the urban world itself creates demands. After my assistant began to work for me (Americans are known to comprise a class of wealthy people), he began receiving demands for money from his father, whom he had not heard from since his parents divorced many years ago. I was paying him a handsome salary by Sierra Leonean standards—a salary level he and I tried to keep secret. But the sudden onslaught of demands from a number of people left him almost penniless after the project finished.

And whereas a foster child may not reciprocate in later years, potential guardians simply may not be given the child they believe themselves entitled to, by virtue of rules of kinship. African kinship systems collapse many relationships into a few classificatory categories. That is, many people are potentially one's "mother," "uncle" or "granny." This plethora of classificatory, not to mention fictive, relatives mean that the actual number of potential foster children rarely matches the array of qualified caretakers. In one neighborhood, several elderly women who had been quite prolific found it hard to obtain any children to foster. In contrast, a nearby barren woman continually fostered at least four small "grandchildren" at a time, using older foster children to help with the younger ones. The factors that seemed to explain her popularity as a guardian were that, unlike her uneducated, poor neighbors, she was an educated business woman and an important member of a powerful family.

If neither fosterage nor biological fertility guarantee support for adults, why do adults want to bear or foster children? I argue that they create levers for adults to lobby for support, using as idioms of persuasion their relationships or assistance to the children. Adults must continually create or shore up obligations, restating their rights, persuading, and even exaggerating their past contributions to the children's upbringing (see also Bates 1975:361). Therefore, rather than speaking of rights in children, the traditional anthropological phraseology, the better way to characterize adults' relationships to children is "claims," which must be created as well as activated. Berry's paper (1987) on Nigerians' efforts to invest in tree crop echoes identical concerns:

> Individuals' access to tree crop farms has depended more on their ability to exercise their claims vis a vis those of other rightholders, than on the way in which they acquired their rights in the first place. . . .

This is not to trivialize children by comparing them to trees, but to stress that the emphasis on future claims, rather than on historically and socially immutable rights, is appropriate in both cases.

Our usual tendency, of course, is to separate children from the messy business of politics—in the sense of negotiated social life—and relegate them safely to the amity of "kinship" with its clear moral expectations. Yet the Mende case places children, fosterage and fertility at the heart of relationships of a surprisingly contractual nature—one that cannot be divorced from power or influence.[4] When taken to its logical conclusion, this perspective blurs the line between parents versus guardians, and that between contract versus moral duty. Instead of carving the world into parents versus guardians, applying wholly different criteria to the two categories, we should view both as investors who must continue perpetually to assert claims on children after the initial fosterage or fertility event.

This approach to reproduction treats fertility and reproduction as a process that can be shaped by intelligent action. The Mende have a saying—"for tomorrow" (*sina va*)—that reflects this in a more general sense. It bespeaks a clear future orientation: a concern with future uncertainty, on the one hand, and, on the other, with plans and strategies to meet future contingencies. Even more important, "for tomorrow" reflects not a passive acceptance of ascribed statuses, but a need to actively shape the future. That is, actions performed today with respect to reproduction are less important for making immediate claims than for laying a basis for future ones.

Conclusion: Socially Constructing Reproduction

Biological parenthood is one way to try to secure later support. But family structure is as much a social and political outcome as a biological one. Although biological fertility does influence how families grow and change, it has limited responsiveness for individuals' changing needs at different life stages. Since Mende methods of family formation are predominantly post-natal and socially managed, customary demographic "cost and benefit" calculuses of biological fertility have little meaning in daily life. Adults continually reassess children and try to adjust their relationships to them, investing more in children who begin to show promise of success and avoiding obligations to those headed for failure. Even parents view a child as a bundle of potentialities, and they treat the original fertility event as the beginning of a long, continuously negotiated relationship (see also Comaroff and Roberts 1981 on the notion of potentialities), a process which competes with simultaneous efforts of other people to lay claims on the same children as investments against unforeseen future circumstances. Because of this, parents would be foolish to outline at the outset of their reproductive careers a clear fertility limitation strategy.

The notion of shaping relationships for the future and the contractual nature of fertility and fosterage stretch the social nature of reproduction to a more flexible and dynamic view, what we might call the "social construction of demographic reality." This approach stresses the fundamental ambiguity of biological and fosterage relations, highlighting people's active efforts to achieve demographic outcomes by restructuring household compositions and influencing children's obligations, rather than acting strictly within the biological bounds or cultural norms that seem to be imposed on them. Individuals constantly tinker with family structures in ways that cumbersome biological acts of fertility cannot.

Notes

1. Alternative approaches—e.g., Caldwell 1978, 1982; Caldwell and Caldwell 1987; Fapohunda 1978; Cain 1981—have sought to expand the analysis to individuals outside the nuclear household.
2. I depart from standard approaches that distinguish between patrons and kin (e.g., Mair 1962). Mende patrons generally turn quickly into kin, as when women are given to powerful men who thereby assume the role of protectors for the donor families (see Murphy and Bledsoe 1987).
3. For fostering out children, other significant associations for women were less education, younger age at first pregnancy, working outside the home, being polygynously married, being Christian, and having more children fostered in. For fostering in children, other significant associations were being older, having some education, not working outside the home, being married, being monogamous, being a migrant, and having more children fostered out. See Antoine and Guillaume (1984) and Findley and Diallo (1988) for discussions of fosterage and fertility. See Ainsworth (1988) for a discussion of the relationship of fosterage to child labor demands.
4. This approach to Mende fosterage and parent-child relations parallels descriptions of ritual *compadrazgo* (godparenthood) in Europe and Latin America (Mintz and Wolf 1950) and *komstvo* in the Balkans (Hammel 1968) in the sense that all of these crystallize immediate obligations where diffuse ones existed before.

References Cited

Ainsworth, Martha. 1988. Child Fostering and the Demand for Child Labor in Côte d'Ivoire. Unpublished manuscript.
Antoine, Philippe, and Agnes Guillaume. 1984. Une Expression de la Solidarite Familiale en Abidjan: Enfants du Couple et Enfants Confies. Les Familles d'Aujourd'hui. Paris: Association International des Demographes de Langue Francais.
Bates, Robert H. 1975. Rural Development in Kasumpa Village, Zambia. Journal of African Studies 2:333–62.
Berry, Sara. 1987. Property Rights and Rural Resource Management: the Case of Tree Crops in West Africa. Working Papers in African Studies, No. 122, African Studies Center, Boston University.
Bledsoe, Caroline. 1980a. The Manipulation of Kpelle Social Fatherhood. Ethnology 19:29–45.
———. 1980b. Women and Marriage in Kpelle Society. Stanford: Stanford University.

———. 1983. Stealing Food as a Problem in Demography and Nutrition. Paper for the 1983 meetings of the American Anthropological Association. Washington, D.C.

———. MS. The Politics of Polygyny in Mende Education and Child Fosterage Transactions. *In* Gender Hierarchies. Barbara Miller, ed.

Bledsoe, Caroline H. and Kenneth M. Robey. 1986. Arabic Literacy and Secrecy among the Mende of Sierra Leone. Man (N.S.) 21:202–226.

Bledsoe, Caroline, Douglas C. Ewbank and Uche C. Isiugo-Abanihe. MS. The Effect of Child Fosterage on Feeding Practices and Access to Health Services in Rural Sierra Leone.

Cain, Mead. 1981. Risk and Insurance: Perspectives on Fertility and Agrarian Change in India and Bangladesh. Population and Development Review 7:435–74.

———. 1982. Perspectives on Family and Fertility in Developing Countries. Population Studies 36:159–175.

Caldwell, John. 1977. The Economic Rationality of High Fertility: An Investigation Illustrated with Nigerian Survey Data. Population Studies 31:5–27.

———. 1978. A Theory of Fertility: From High Plateau to Destabilization. Population and Development Review 4:553-77.

———. 1982. Theory of Fertility Decline. New York: Academic Press.

Caldwell, John C. and Pat Caldwell. 1987. The Cultural Context of High Fertility in Sub-Saharan Africa. Population and Development Review 13:409–37.

Comaroff, John L. and Simon Roberts. 1981. Rules and Processes: The Cultural Logic of Dispute in an African Context. Chicago: University of Chicago.

Etienne, Mona. 1983. Gender Relations and Conjugality among the Baule. *In* Female and Male in West Africa. Christine Oppong, ed. Pp. 303–319. London: George Allen and Unwin.

Fapohunda, Eleanor. 1978. Characteristics of Women Workers in Lagos. Labour and Society 3:158–171.

Findley, Sally E., and Assitan Diallo. 1988. Foster Children: Links Between Urban and Rural Families? Proceedings of the Second African Population Conference, Volume 2, Dakar, Senegal.

Frank, Odile. 1984. Child-fostering in Sub-Saharan Africa. Presentation for the Population Association of America. Minneapolis, Minn.

Goody, Esther N. 1982. Parenthood and Social Reproduction: Fostering and Occupational Roles in West Africa.Cambridge: Cambridge University.

Goody, Jack. 1971. Class and marriage in Africa and Eurasia. American Journal of Sociology 76:585–603.

Hammel, Eugene A. 1968. Alternative Social Structures and Ritual Relations in the Balkans. Englewood Cliffs, N.J.: Prentice-Hall.

Handwerker, W. Penn. 1987. Fiscal Corruption and the Moral Economy of Resource Acquisition. Research in Economic Anthropology 9:307–353.

Isaac, Barry R. & Shelby R. Conrad. 1982. Child Fosterage among the Mende of Upper Bambara Chiefdom, Sierra Leone: Rural-urban and Occupational Comparisons. Ethnology 21:243–257.

Isiugo-Abanihe, Uche. 1985. Child Fosterage in West Africa. Population and Development Review 11:53–73.

Kopytoff, Igor and Suzanne Miers. 1977. Introduction. *In* Slavery in Africa: Historical and Anthropological Perspectives. Igor Kopytoff and Suzanne Miers, eds. Pp. 3-81. Madison: University of Wisconsin.

Mintz, S.W. and E.R. Wolf. 1950. An Analysis of Ritual Co-parenthood (Compadrazgo). Southwestern Journal of Anthropology 6:341-365.

Murphy, William P. 1981. The Rhetorical Management of Dangerous Knowledge as Property and Power in Kpelle Brokerage. American Ethnologist 8:667-685.

Murphy, William P. and Caroline H. Bledsoe. 1987. Kinship and Territory in the History of a Kpelle Chiefdom (Liberia). *In* The African Frontier: The Reproduction of Traditional African Societies. Igor Kopytoff, ed. Pp. 121-147. Bloomingtom: Indiana University.

Okore, Augustine. 1977. The Ibos of Arochukwu in Imo State, Nigeria. *In* The Persistence of High Fertility. John C.Caldwell, ed. Pp. 313-329. Canberra: Australian National University.

Oppong, Christine. 1973. Growing Up in Dagbon. Accra.

Oppong, Christine and Wolf Bleek. 1982. Economic Models and Having Children: Some Evidence from Kwahu, Ghana. Africa 52:15-33.

Page, Hilary J. (in press). Child-rearing versus Child-bearing: Co-residence of Mother and Children in Sub-Saharan Africa. *In* Ronald J.Lesthaeghe, ed. African Reproduction and Social Organization. Berkeley: University of California Press.

Scheper-Hughes, Nancy, ed. 1987. Child Survival: Anthropological Perspectives on the Treatment and Maltreatment of Children. D. Reidel.

Schildkrout, Enid. 1973. The Fostering of Children in Urban Ghana: Problems of Ethnographic Analysis in a Multi-cultural Context. Urban Anthropology 2:48-73.

Scrimshaw, Susan C. W. 1978. Infant Mortality and Behavior in the Regulation of Family Size. Population and Development Review 4:383-403.

Sembajwe, I.S.L. 1977. Socio-cultural Supports for High Fertility in Buganda. *In* The Economic and Social Supports for Higher Fertility. Lado T.Ruzicka, ed. Pp. 135-151. Canberra: Australian National University

Thomas, Armand C. 1983. The Population of Sierra Leone: An Analysis of Population Census Data. Freetown: Demographic Research and Training Unit, Fourah Bay College.

6

The Politics of Below-Replacement Fertility: Policy and Power in Hungary

Jeanne M. Simonelli

While much of the world attempts to slow population growth, Hungarian policy is designed to stimulate births by using broad economic and social incentives. In a country of long-standing low fertility, women responded to the program by altering birth timing and spacing without increasing completed family size. Examination of the historical and contemporary circumstances surrounding the fertility decisions of women and couples in socialist Hungary reveals a complex relationship between women's rights, production, and reproduction. This chapter examines that relationship by briefly outlining the characteristics of the demographic transition in Eastern Europe, relating fertility decline to the productive needs of post World War II Hungary and, finally, through an analysis of the interaction of social, economic, and demographic policy in contemporary Hungary. These multidimensional forces, which produced the current structure of Hungarian population, have often been in opposition. Societal goals did not always correspond with the hopes and dreams of individuals, whose own decisions concerning childbearing often go beyond the practical and obvious, and into the realm of the emotional and nonquantifiable.

Prologue:
The Demographic Transition in Eastern Europe

Eastern Europe experienced a demographic transition which differed from that occurring in western and northern Europe. Beginning about fifty years later than in the latter areas, the transitionary period lacked the typical "European marriage pattern" (Hajnal 1965) of delayed and non-universal marriage with high marital fertility. Instead, by the middle of the nineteenth century, Eastern Europe was characterized by an extraordinarily high proportion of marriage in the population, with only moderate levels of fertility within the marriage. This marked a change from a pattern of early marriage and uncontrolled fertility to one in which fertility control was becoming prevalent (Barta et al. 1985; David and McIntyre 1981).

In an attempt to explain why fertility is controlled within marriage some researchers, drawing on Habbakuk (1955) and Hajnal (1965), point to the relationship between inheritance patterns and industrialization as key variables. Those studying Western Europe concluded that im-partible inheritance patterns lowered nuptiality and fertility rates because only one individual per family could inherit. This is said to have produced slower demographic growth than did partible inheritance patterns in which all offspring received a small stake with which to begin marriage and child bearing (Thompson 1983). In contrast, Hungarian demographers have asserted that partible inheritance led to lower fertility in Hungary, in spite of continued early marriage (Cseh-Szombathy 1983). There, land for cultivation was already severely limited by the mid-eighteenth century. Because it was necessary to divide the amount of production capacity and goods between all family members, Hungarians chose to limit not only fertility, but also the number of children who survived to adulthood (Andorka 1978:94-95). Evidence for this has been found in early eth-nographies and sociographies, which are rich with supportive quotations.

> We do not make beggars. The country is full of unemployed people. There are more people than would be necessary. What do you want from us? Give us land and the land will produce children (Andorka 1978:95).

This attitude produced specific cultural norms which mandated fertility limitation.

> If a married woman remained sterile, she was sympathized with; if she had no living children, it was said "it is her concern;" but if she had more than two children, she was ridiculed, despised, condemned—"Can she not take care?" or "I would be ashamed if I littered as much"—and the mother or mother-in-law generally knew the proper time to recommend "It is better to wash the sheeting than the baby's napkin (Andorka 1978:95)."

According to these accounts, when fertility control was not effective, neglect-based infanticide occurred.

This pattern did not pertain throughout the entire country, but was related to the type of agricultural activity in an area. Small-holders had much more interest in limiting their fertility than did agricultural laborers working the large estates of landlords (cf. Handwerker 1986; Schneider and Schneider 1984). In spite of this variation, fertility in Hungary achieved only moderate levels compared to other countries in Europe. At the turn of the century, for example, Hungarian women were bearing children at a rate which would have given them just over 5 children, on average, by the end of their reproductive career.

Figure 6.1 displays Hungarian fertility trends over the course of the 20th century as measured by the Net Reproduction Rate. The Net Reproduction Rate measures women's ability to replace themselves and, thus, to generate long-term population growth or decline. An NRR of 2.00 means that each woman replaces herself with two daughters and that the population doubles in size each generation. An NRR of 1.00 means that each woman replaces herself with exactly one daughter and that the population neither grows nor declines. An NRR below 1.00 means that women have so few children that they do not even replace themselves, and that the population grows smaller with each subsequent generation. (An NRR of .5 means that the population will be reduced by one-half each generation unless immigration offsets the population decline.)

Figure 6.1 shows that Hungarian fertility declined markedly during World War I, and fell below replacement level during the subsequent world depression and World War II. Fertility rose dramatically during the stability and improving economic conditions which followed World War II, particularly through the early 1950s when antiabortion laws were rigidly enforced. Hungarian fertility fell equally dramatically to below replacement levels once access to abortion was liberalized. Fertility rose slightly when the government instituted its pro-natalist policy and began to restrict access to abortion. This rise was temporary, however. By the late 1970s, Hungarian women were again bearing fewer than 2 children, on average, over the course of their reproductive careers, and fertility has remained below replacement levels since that time. The rest of this chapter explains why and how Hungarian women have thwarted government attempts to raise their fertility.

Agriculture, Economy, and Demographic Policy in Post-WWII Hungary

The experience of the last forty years has taught official Hungary that women do, indeed, stand at the crossroads of reproductive and productive behavior. As one of the lesser developed countries of Europe at the close of World War II, the nation was faced with completing industrialization. The process of rapid conversion to heavy industry was

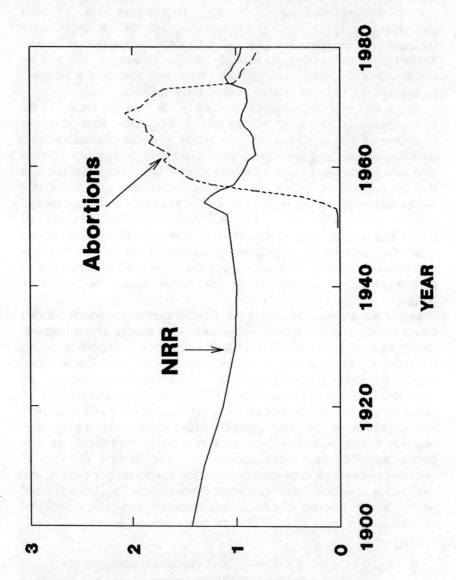

NRR and No. of Abortions (000,000s)

FIGURE 6.1 Net Reproduction Rate (NRR) and Number of Abortions for Hungary, 1900–1980. *Source:* David and McIntyre (1981, Tables 12.1 and 12.3).

characterized by a substitution of labor intensive methods for missing skills and technology. To meet these needs, in socialist Hungary the right to work became a legal obligation. Although married women were not compelled to work, the wage structure was kept artificially low, and families required two wage-earners to maintain a decent living standard (Ferge 1978:89).

In Socialist countries the commitment to equality of the sexes is ideological in origin. Women cannot have equal status with men unless they are participants in social and economic activity (Anker 1985:1). With this in mind, Hungarian women were granted instant liberation following World War II. Because short term industrial needs required that women work, not much attention was paid to the country's long term labor requirements which could only be met through reproduction. Marxist ideology had proclaimed the equality of women without bothering to work out certain of the practical issues related to that equality (Scott 1974:117–163).

One such issue is that women found new opportunities to escape economic dependence on their husbands and their children. As the process of development accelerated through the 1950s, childbearing became increasingly disadvantageous. By the late 1950s, Hungarians were bearing children at a rate which would have given them just over 2 children, on average, at the end of their reproductive career, a number insufficient for the replacement of the population.

Behind the scenes, demographers and social scientists were not alarmed by this, stating that the decline represented a cohort effect of previous lows and was entirely precedented given Hungary's reproductive history. Moreover, there was some fear that the country's nonproductive infrastructure, including hospitals and child care facilities, could not support population growth. In contrast, economists were distressed, since they associated declining birth rates with women's employment. They viewed the loss of reproductive potential as capable of producing a future labor shortage (cf. Lapidus 1978:92). State ideologues were caught in the middle, faced with violating dogma by removing women from the workforce in order to utilize their reproductive capacities. In addition, recognition of Hungary's long term needs meant disregarding the short term demands of labor and industry. The solution to this problem was provided by still another group of actors. This group, dubbed the "Literary nationalists" by demographers on the opposing side, was comprised of a number of prominent, respected writers.

In the aftermath of the 1956 revolution, Hungarian society was in need of a revitalizing and unifying force (cf. Thorton 1981). These writers saw the demographic issue as providing a means to this end. By proclaiming Hungary to be on the brink of extinction, they appealed to the nationalistic, non-partisan sentiments of both policymakers and the populace in devising a comprehensive plan aimed at altering the reproductive behavior of Hungarian couples. The final result of this campaign was a broad program of family policy characterized by monetary and in-kind incentives for increasing births. A key element was the possibility of subsidized long term care for preschool children at home (program benefits are listed in the Appendix).

During the years 1967 to 1973 demographic policy was limited to the provision of direct and indirect incentives to families with children. In 1973, the scope of the program was extended into the social and moral spheres as well. Compulsory instruction in family planning and birth timing was introduced. Health education programs were added to the school curricula. Regulations to reduce the number of induced abortions were instituted. In 1975, provisions granting time off to nursing mothers and extensive paid leave for care of sick children also became part of the benefit package (Hungarian Review 1979:6; Szabady 1978:90–91).

Though certain of these benefits were available to unmarried women, many were implicitly designed to encourage marriage. The core of the program remains the child care allowance. An economically active mother who remains on child care leave is entitled to this benefit until the child is aged three. In 1982 it became legally possible for the father to remain at home with the child and receive the allowance. In 1985, demographic policy prompted expenditures of about nine percent of the net national product on programs including family allowances, maternity benefits, child care allowances, nursing, and sick pay (Barta et al. 1985). It is important to note that by 1983, Hungarian family policy had become a social program critical to the legitimization of the political system. Demographers who had opposed the program were forced to admit that regardless of demographic impact, the country was irreversibly committed to maintaining all aspects (Cseh-Szombathy 1983).

The Changing Demands of the Hungarian Economy

Beginning in 1968, the Hungarian government attempted to break out of socialist patterns of inefficient industrial production by reform and decentralization of the economy. Between 1968 and 1972, the GNP showed a steady increase and the standard of living began to rise. Economists were determined to build an economically rational system in which the market mechanism and efficient production dominated regardless of who owned the means of production. Hungarian prices became tied to those of the world market, and hard currency exports to the West were pushed to their limits (Bacskai 1983; N.Y. Times 1986).

In time it became evident that efficiency (and profit) could not be achieved if the prevailing pattern of under-employment persisted. Although labor shortages did exist in skilled and semi-skilled areas, by the mid-seventies there was a surplus of unskilled and manual laborers. As a result, the economists began to argue that there was a rational need for unemployment. In contrast, social scientists argued that the legitimacy of the State was derived from the maintenance of the socialist social compact guaranteeing full employment, as well as social programs and an increasing standard of living. Hungarian wages were still kept artificially low, necessitating more than one income from more than one source. As a partial response to this dilemma, the government relaxed controls on private economic activity, particularly in the agricultural sector. Individuals resumed market gardening and animal husbandry, activities that were the domain of women traditionally. Within a short time, five percent of Hungarian land was producing thirty percent of agricultural goods, much of which would ultimately be exported for hard currency. A worker could earn eighty to one hundred percent of his/her yearly wage in this "second economy" sector. Consumers were able to earn the money to satisfy their demand for consumer goods by working on household plots (Csaki 1983). The second economy became essential for Hungarian prosperity, functioning in areas not represented in the regular economy. Private enterprise stayed operative at high levels because regular wages remained depressed, creating a need for additional income. Women who remained at home on the childcare allowance were able to use that time to work in market gardens, thus supplementing regular wage income in two ways (Simonelli 1985).

By 1982, Hungary was faced with an ideological and practical crisis. They had developed a massive and expensive program of family policy in response to a misinterpreted demographic problem; they were faced with a surplus of unskilled workers, especially in those areas which traditionally employed women; and they had to maintain an active, private second economy in order to preserve the country's economic and psychological well-being. Three issues, motherhood, unemployment, and private enterprise became critical to maintaining socialism in Hungary, yet all three seriously violated the ideological basis for Hungarian society. The key to the resolution of this problem was women—who found increasing opportunities to make choices on the basis of what was best for themselves, in spite of the machinations of those in control on a societal level.

In 1987 participation in the private agricultural economy became an even more lucrative and essential activity for Hungarian households. In the wake of increasing economic problems, the government imposed a new program of personal income taxes which touched all aspects of earning except the income of private farmers. Consequently, the incentive to remain at home and farm was even greater than had been previously (Economist 1987).

The Impact of Demographic Policy

All measures that were introduced to manipulate the birth rate in Hungary produced little or no population growth, as apparent in Figure 1. Although periods of short term increase were seen, each instance was immediately followed by a down trend. The greatest upsurge in births occurred from 1974-1976. This followed the 1973 policy modifications cited above, including restrictions on induced abortions. According to Hungarian analysis of the data, population policy has had a greater impact on the *timing* of births than on completed family size. Because birth incentives provided greater financial security, families who would have eventually had two children were willing to have the second child earlier than previously planned (Barta et al. 1985; Klinger 1977:168).

Although state-instituted demographic policy was unable to modify the overall Hungarian fertility picture, individual aspects of the program have left an indelible mark on the structure of Hungarian society. Moreover, the behavior of Hungarian women in utilizing family allowances sheds some light on the decision-making process for women in advanced societies.

In 1979, it was estimated that 250,000 women were at home on child care allowances (Barta et al. 1985; Hungarian Review 1979:22). In 1977, the ratio of those utilizing these subsidies to the number of children in state nurseries was four to one. It was estimated that 90 percent of all births satisfied eligibility criteria for the allowances, and 80 percent of these actually made use of them (Huszar and Suranyi 1980:131). In a non-government study, Coelen and McIntyre concluded that 13 percent of eligible women would stay home even if no monetary reimbursement were involved. They calculated that because of the subsidy, 52 percent of eligibles were actually doing so (1978:1077–1099).

Studies conducted in the years following the establishment of the allowance stated that the decision to give up work and social connections, or to remain a working mother, reflected the nature of a woman's occupation. Manually employed women chose to stay at home, as did clerical workers. Those engaged in professions with higher earnings were less likely to chance a break in their careers. Educational background also influenced the decision to stay home. Seventy-two percent of women with elementary education, 60 percent of those with secondary education, and 30 percent of those with advanced education utilized the leave (Szabady 1977:380–399). According to Ferge (1983), this use of the child care allowance by unskilled women effectively removed four percent of the total work force from competition for employment. This pleased the economists who continued to maintain that Hungary must find other ways to encourage women to remain at home and resume reproductive activities.

Until recently, Hungarian women were reluctant to interrupt careers because status was tied to profession. However, as a result of the second economy, material living conditions now also determine an individual's place in the social system. For many, it is the status value of material goods rather than the joys of motherhood that has influenced the reproductive decisions of Hungarian women. If this is the case then it is the convergence of monetary rewards associated with both childbearing and the agriculturally-based second economy that has influenced the change in birth spacing for Hungarian women. As Handwerker noted, variation in fertility is accounted for by behavioral change following from demand for an adequate and reliable flow of income (1983, 1986).

In Hungary today, women are still utilizing a strategy of low marital fertility that had its basis in the historic evaluation of scarce resources related to land available for subsistence. In a sense, the Hungarian government has tried to assume the role of the virile mate by attempting to increase its social reproductive success by convincing women to have more than their optimal number of children. Hungarian women, however, continue to assess resources as scarce and, while appearing to alter their strategies, do not really do so. The flow of income, in the form of positive monetary incentives provided by the state, was not deemed sufficiently reliable to cause an ultimate increase in total fertility rates. In the absence of social system changes, short term monetary incentives produced only short term change.

Appendix: Benefit Provisions of Hungarian Population Policy

Maternity Grant/Childbirth Allowance: Payable to all women who have worked within 6 months of the pregnancy or are covered by social insurance, as long as the mother has at least one pre-natal consultation prior to the birth. The amount is 2500 forint per child, or about 3/4 of the average monthly wage.

Maternity Allowance/Pregnancy Confinement Grant: Payable to all women who have been insured for six months in the two years before confinement. Full pay, payable for 20 weeks. May be extended in the case of problem pregnancies.

Family Allowance: This is paid monthly to all parents with two or more children under the age of 16, and for 3 more years if the children are still in school. Payable for one child in the case of disadvantaged parents or children.

Sick Pay: If the child is under the age of one, it is payable indefinitely. For a child aged 1-3 years it is payable for 60 days, and for those 3-6 years for 30 days. Available to the mother or the father.

Nursing Mothers: Nursing mothers who return to work after the regular 20 week leave and continue to nurse their babies are entitled to one hour off per day for the first two months and 1/2 hour per day for the next two months.

Loan and Apartment Preference: Young married couples with families are given preference in receiving loans to be used toward purchasing apartments or homes, as well as priorities on waiting lists for the above housing.

Child Care Allowance: This is the most crucial allowance for the mother wishing to chose between returning to work or staying at home with her infant. It is payable to any mother until her child reaches the age of three, providing that the mother has been working for a period longer than a term pregnancy prior to that birth. If she is married her husband must also be employed. Years spent at home do not constitute a break in employment and on her return to work, wages are adjusted as if she had never been away. Payable to fathers, and for more than one child at a time.

References Cited

Anker, R. 1985. Comparative Survey. *In* Working Women in Socialist Countries. Bodrova. V. and Anker R. eds. Pp. 1–21. Geneva: International Labour Office.

Andorka, R. 1978. Determinants of Fertility in Advanced Societies. New York: The Free Press.

Bacskai, T. 1983. Hungarian Economic Policy. Presented at the 1983 Social Science Seminar in Debrecen, Hungary. July 20–21, 1983.

Barta, Barnabas, Andras Klinger, Karoly Miltenyi, and Gyorgy Vukovich. 1985. Female Labour Force Participation and Fertility in Hungary. *In* Working Women in Socialist Countries. Bodrova, V. and Anker, R. eds. Pp. 23–53. Geneva: International Labour Office.

Coelen, S.P. and R.J. McIntyre. 1978. An Econometric Model of Pronatalist and Abortion Policies. Journal of Political Economy 86(6):1077–1099.

Csaki, C. 1983. Features of Present Day Hungarian Agricultural Economy. Presented at the 1983 Social Science Seminar in Debrecen, Hungary, July 27, 1983.

Cseh-Szombathy, L. 1983. The Hungarian Family. Presented at the 1983 Social Science Seminar in Debrecen, Hungary.

David, H.P. and R.J. McIntyre. 1981. Reproductive Behavior: Central and Eastern European Experience. New York: Springer Publishing Company.

Economist. 1987. Hungary: Taxing Times. Sept. 12, 1987. p. 54.

Ferge, Z. 1980 . A Society in the Making: Hungarian Social and Societal Policy 1945-1975. White Plains, New York: M.E. Sharp, Inc.

––––––. 1983. Societal Policy: Social Structural Concerns. Presented at the Social Science Seminar in Debrecen, Hungary. August 1, 1983.

Habakkuk, H.J. 1955. Family Structure and Economic Change in Nineteenth-Century Europe. The Journal of Economic History. XV(1):1–12.

Hajnal, J. 1965. European Marriage Patterns in Perspective. *In* Population in History. D.V. Glass and Eversley eds. Pp. 101–146. London: Edward Arnold.

Handwerker, W.P. 1983. The First Demographic Transition: An Analysis of Subsistence Choices and Reproductive Consequences. American Anthropologist 84(1):5–27.

———. 1986. The Modern Demographic Transition: An Analysis of Subsistence Choices and Reproductive Consequences. American Anthropologist 88(2):400–417.

Hungarian Review. 1979. Providing for the Child. Vol. 6.

Huszar, M. and B. Suranyi. 1980. The Employment of Women in Hungary. New Hungarian Quarterly 2:125–132.

Klinger, A. 1977. Fertility and Family Planning in Hungary. Studies in Family Planning. 8:166–176.

Lapidus, G. 1978. Women in Soviet Society. Berkeley: University of California Press.

New York Times. 1986. Budapest: Making A Forint–Ideology and a Bit of Free Enterprise. March 23, p. 41.

Schneider, J. and P. Schneider. 1984. Demographic Transitions in a Sicilian Rural Town. Journal of Family History 9:245–272.

Scott, H. 1974. Does Socialism Liberate Women? Experiences From Eastern Europe. Boston: Beacon Press.

Simonelli, J.M. 1985. The Entrepreneuring Village: (or How Much Produce can a Peasant Producer Produce if a Peasant Producer Profits from Production?). Journal of Anthropology 4(1).

Szabadyk, Egon. 1977. Impact of the New Child Care Allowances. *In* Modern Hungary. D. Sinor, ed. Bloomington: Indiana University Press.

———. 1978. Family Centered Population Policy in Hungary. New Hungarian Quarterly 3:87–93.

Thompson, S.I. 1983. Inheritance Patterns and Industrialization in China and Japan. Paper presented at the annual meeting of Society for applied Anthropology. Toronto, Canada, March, 1984.

Thorton, R. 1981. Demographic Antecedents of a Revitalization Movement: Population Change, Population Size, and the 1890 Ghost Dance. American Sociology Review 46:88–96.

7

The Politics of Parenthood: Fairness, Freedom, and Responsibility in American Reproductive Choices

Catherine L. Leone

The prevailing political philosophy of the United States as a nation is individualism, which holds that the interests of the individual are or ought to be ethically paramount, and that all values, rights, and duties originate in individuals. This doctrine maintains the political and economic independence of the individual and stresses individual initiative, action, and interests. With deep roots in British history and posed in the rhetoric of Enlightenment philosophers, the principles of individualism are codified in the Constitution and the Bill of Rights, and reinforced generation after generation by a system of universal public education.

Although we are most familiar with the way Locke, Mill, and Jefferson, for example, articulate the rights and responsibilities of individuals, individualism predates the 18th century. Macfarlane (1978) traces individualism back to the 14th century in England, noting that even at this early date, English men and women held property as individuals, not as families. Macfarlane's work establishes the central role of individualism in English institutions hundreds of years earlier than previously thought. To the extent that American institutions, from law and government to marriage and kinship, are modeled on the British example, we share an extremely old and powerful legacy.

In the United States, historians, political scientists, sociologists, and anthropologists have, with varying emphasis, pointed to this constellation of values and propositions about the nature of human beings to explain a variety of social phenomena, and in doing so confirm its central place in American thought and behavior. For example, in his history of the American family (1980), Degler recounts how the very logic of individualism called for its extension to women (e.g., Mill's 1869 tract, *The*

Subjection of Women) and to nonwhites, despite the fact that the "individuals" to whom Enlightenment writers refer are exclusively male. In particular, he calls our attention to the role of individualism in the transformation of the 19th century family in America from a patriarchal, economic institution to the modern, child-centered, affectively oriented family. Addressing a very different question, Hochschild (1981) examines the role of American ideas about democracy and justice across all socioeconomic classes. Using material from an exhaustive interview schedule of open-ended questions, she concludes that the American penchant for procedural, as opposed to distributive, justice explains the lack of success of the socialist movement in this country. Hsu, long involved in national character studies, argues that the many seemingly contradictory values espoused by Americans are manifestations of one core value, self-reliance, which has its roots in the British demand for political equality. In America, this insistence on inalienable political rights of the individual is expanded and has become inseparable from the individual's militant insistence on unlimited economic, social, and political equality, finding its most extreme manifestation in the American obsession with political equality as a right and individualism as the "natural" state of man (Hsu 1972).

It is clear that individualistic principles play a large role in Americans' perception of the political process and in the day-to-day interactions of people with their institutions at all levels. Might these principles be expected to play a major role in women's reasoning about the personal decision to reproduce? Witness the dramatic changes for women since the 1950s: Women currently are marrying later, which allows them more time to establish economic and social independence before marriage. Women are divorcing and remarrying at higher rates. The proportion of female household heads has increased dramatically, and a significant number of these are women with dependent children. More women are earning college and advanced degrees, most in traditionally female fields. Labor force participation of women is much greater although, like women's education, it continues to be concentrated in only a few occupations (Bianchi and Spain 1986). In a remarkable turnaround from the years of the baby boom, fertility has fallen to levels far below replacement and shows no propensity to rise above that level.

This chapter shows that, in a new context created by changes in the status of women, individualism and its associated values have become integral elements of the choices American women make to have or not to have children. I have found that three such values, fairness, freedom, and responsibility, are crucial in the reasoning surrounding women's reproductive decision making. Further, examination of how these values are acted out clarifies the connections between reproductive decisions at the individual level and fertility trends at the national level.

Methods and Data

This analysis is based on interviews with 31 women in Washington State conducted between 1980 and 1983 (Leone 1986). Informant selection, data collection, and analysis were designed to discover motivations for reproduction among middle-class American women and the factors that enter into the decision-making process. Twenty study participants were mothers; 11 were childless at the time of the interview. Both mothers and currently childless women were included in order to capitalize on the findings of Cooper et al. (1978:81) who report that childless wives experience "intense questioning of their motives and a need to justify their decision to others." It was hoped that the testimony of childless women would provide meaningful contrast with the possibly less explicit reasoning of women who had chosen to have children, a behavior for which there is less need of legitimizing explanations.

Despite some differences, the mothers and nonmothers in the study are quite similar with regard to age, education, marital status and history, and family background. The study population displays a consistent pattern of higher levels of education, later age at marriage, and later age at childbirth than American women on average. As a group, they embody all of the major trends which characterize changes in women's status over the past 40 years.

In open-ended interviews, all informants were asked about their reasons for having, postponing, or not having children. Transcripts of the interviews were then analyzed for the presence and relative importance of 20 motivational and conditioning factors. These factors were derived from my participation for several months in group discussions with the women of a parent-child cooperative, from the preliminary review of the interview data, and from the literature on fertility motivation, especially Gabriel's study of reproductive motivation (1983). These 20 factors represent a wide range of circumstances and motives that seem likely to affect the decision to have children. They were used to direct the review of the transcribed interviews.

Findings in Brief

Findings from the interviews can be summarized in terms of motivations and ideal prerequisites for parenthood, and general rules for reproductive decisions. Informant statements about primary family relationships showed that motives for reproduction are expressed largely in terms of nuclear family relationships. The consensus among the informants is that the primary motive for motherhood is a desire for the relationship with one's own child, and that there is a set of prerequisites for parenthood, which are variations on the themes of emotional and financial stability. The most important and most highly approved motive for childbearing is a desire for a child to love and care for. This finding is supported at the population level by survey research on the value of children in developed countries (e.g., Fawcett 1978, Bulatao 1981). This affective motive for childbearing tends to characterize low-fertility, industrialized societies, where economic incentives for having children are low or nonexistent. Women's discussions of the relevance of their age, economic situation, career aspirations, and family goals to child-bearing decisions provide a picture of ideal prerequisites for parenthood.

The literature on reproductive decision making and fertility trends is dominated by quantitative research on nationally representative data sets. Given that, it is reassuring that in-depth interviews with a small (minute by statistical standards) group of women corroborates survey research, with regard to the importance of personal autonomy and responsibility in the decision-making process and with regard to the more frequently cited motives for childbearing. Beyond such mutual validation, it is crucial to note that an ethnographic approach allows release from the constraints of survey research and discovery of new ideas about how women shape their reproductive decisions. The concept of fairness occurs in the interview data so often and in such a wide array of contexts, I was led to conclude that this is an extremely important value in reproductive decision making. This new finding, not noted in the sociological literature, is grounded in women's perception of themselves and their children as individuals whose interests must be taken into account.

Freedom and Responsibility

When women consider having children, the freedom of childlessness or of a "child-free lifestyle," is contrasted with the responsibilities of parenthood, which bring as well a sense of adult status, the pleasures and challenges of parent-child interaction, and the symbolic completion of the family which comes with creating a new generation. Given the foregoing discussion of individualism, it is understandable that independence has a high value for Americans and the prospect of reduced independence as children arrive is commonly involved in fertility decisions. From interviews of 44 child-free couples, Cooper et al. report that "Men and women agreed that the most important motive to remain child free was 'more personal freedom'" (1978:76). Drawing from a cross-national study, the Value of Children Project, Fawcett reports that in the United States, "For a question asking how a woman's or a man's life is changed by having children, the most common response category for men and women at all parities was 'restrictions on freedom'" (1978:258).

Coexisting with the tendency to maximize independence is an impetus toward attaining responsibility and adulthood, and having children can represent that attainment. That both independence and responsibility are valued and sought is amply demonstrated in the discourse of my informants. Half of the mothers and over 70 percent of the childless women I interviewed made statements that related balancing freedom and responsibility to fertility decision making. Virtually all these statements support the idea that freedom and independence are limited by having children, and that having children is a significant personal and social responsibility.

For example, childless women report:

In high school, I decided that I didn't want children, because I could see that they would be a tremendous interference in my life and freedom.

The freedom element has always been very important, and I would be unwilling to give it up for children. To have children right now would mean my being out of the work force and unable to pursue any kind of career goals.

Mothers are also aware of the loss of freedom children entail:

I feel really committed to staying home for the first two years of a child's life, at least, that's a given for my value system. And I didn't want to stay home again, tied down. I had been very involved in community activities revolving around my son. I was back in school and enjoying it.

I thought I was ready, but after the child came it really hit me hard, when I realized that I didn't have the opportunity to get out and do things spontaneously like I'd always done before.

Over half of the statements about the limits to independence induced by motherhood were made by childless women, who made up only one-third of the study group, suggesting that the weight placed on personal autonomy as a desired state is greater for women who are currently childless by choice.

That the responsibility imposed by children can be a burden does not escape my informants:

I was a little apprehensive about getting pregnant, mainly because of losing my freedom. And I knew it would fall on me, the responsibility. And any woman that doesn't [realize that] is stupid, in this society.

I felt a lot of responsibility and not a lot of joy and satisfaction in having children around. I have felt very constricted and felt that I took more responsibility for those kids than their father did. I am a more "responsible" person.

Reported changes in behavior, which women associate with parenthood, suggest the all-inclusive nature of the responsibility bestowed on parents. Such behavioral changes include driving more carefully, curtailment of drinking alcohol, retiring from dangerous sports, deleting profanity from the vocabulary, and coming home earlier from social events. These changes may have the practical advantage of safeguarding the child, but they also reinforce the parents' image as proper parents.

At the same time the responsibility of parenthood may be seen as onerous, it is seen as an avenue to adult status and as evidence of maturity:

I think having a child would have helped me a lot in the struggle for separation from my parents. Getting married is one way to separate. Having a child makes it clear that you are making your own decision, and I think that's acknowledged from both sides. So that would have helped me in some ways to become an adult in my mother's eyes.

Our neighbors made their children call me Mrs. Bowden, and that always freaked me out because I was only 20 years old and they were all calling me Mrs. Bowden. It definitely gives you a life, or a status, or whatever you want to call it to have a child in tow.

That reproductive decisions imply responsibility to the community beyond the family is suggested here:

I certainly get the feeling that, in the opinion of this community, you're being irresponsible to the global society if you have more than two children.

The ecological thing. I think the responsible thing is to limit your children to two or three.

It's also irresponsible, that size family [four children], I realize, but for the family itself, I think that's ideal. But there are too many people around. Four is double replacement value. I don't think that kind of ecological reasoning would deter me at all. It might deter my husband, who is really rabid about that.

These statements are telling examples of the individualistic principle that responsibilities as well as rights originate with the individual.

Fairness

According to Webster, to be fair is to be "marked by impartiality and honesty, free from self-interest, prejudice or favoritism" (Webster's *New Collegiate Dictionary*, 1973). Fairness implies an elimination of personal feelings, interests, prejudices so as to achieve a proper balance of conflicting needs, rights, or demands. It is in this sense of striving for balance, equitability, and evenhandedness that women invoke fairness as a guide for behavior and a justification for reproductive decisions and actions. Rather than lacking self-interest, women attempt to address their family planning decisions in such a way that the interests of the "self" are assessed evenly with those of the other parties involved.

It is important to demonstrate the prevalence of the concept of fairness in the interviews. Women allude to fairness in every context addressed in the interview. The recurrence of this theme was surprising to me during the interviewing phase of the research, and again as I reviewed the entire corpus of data. Nothing in the demographic literature suggests that fairness might be a factor. Fairness figures prominently in informants' discussion of providing siblings for an existing child, the advantages and disadvantages of the "only child," quality of care for children, husband's role in reproductive decisions, providing economic security, and balancing work outside the home with child rearing. Other contexts which were discussed less frequently, but in which fairness was cited, include spacing of births, parental lifestyle, potential for birth defects in offspring, families with more than three children, fear of being an inadequate parent, the perception of children as a hedge against want in old age, and whether fertile women should adopt. Thus, the entire spectrum of family planning issues is imbued with the fairness principle. These tend to appear in the interviews as pronouncements about what's not fair. For example: "It's not fair to have an only child," or, "It's not fair to have more children than you can provide for." These are actually personal statements about what is fitting for the life situation of each speaker.

Let us examine some excerpts from the interview data. The informant statements discussed below are taken from the interviews of 17 women, 11 who are mothers and 6 who are childless—a proportion of mothers to childless women representative of the study group as a whole. Both mothers and childless women use the idiom of fairness for discussing their choices in a remarkably similar way.

Fairness is clearly an important consideration for the number of children women desire to have, especially in the context of providing sibling(s) for an existing child or avoiding an "only child" family. The value of having siblings is recognized for both the juvenile and adult stages of life. Ten women made statements on this theme, eight holding the position that it is unfair for the child not to have siblings. Women who express this attitude tend to be unequivocal about it:

> I would like to provide a sibling for my child. On the other hand, I am never going to make a great deal of money. I want to be able to send my children to any college they want to go to. It's hard for me to evaluate how important this sibling is. I'm inclined to think it's pretty important. The only reason I would have a second child is for the child, not for me.

> I just really feel that it's wrong to have only one child. I don't think it's fair to the parents or the child.

> The other reason for wanting another child is just really for our daughter's sake.

> If we could we'd really like to have another one, because I'd like for her not to be an only child, more for her sake, really.

> If you're going to have one, you should at least have two. They need a sibling.

The prevalence of this attitude is indicated by the fact that the woman who made the statement immediately above is herself a divorced mother of an only child and plans to have no other children should she remarry.

One of the ten women who addressed the topic was neutral on the "fairness" of providing siblings; she has heard this idea voiced by other women but feels that having siblings is a matter of indifference to the child. As an example of how hewing to the principle of fairness can lead to different outcomes, the tenth woman holds that it is unfair to the second child to have that second child in order to provide companionship for the first:

> I thought about it a lot and finally thought a child has to be born in and of itself, not because I don't want my first child to be an only child.

The examples above indicate that fairness is invoked to explain reproductive strategies that range from planning large families ("every boy should have a brother, every girl should have a sister") to planning an only child.

The interaction of women with their spouses is another area in which decisions are to be tempered with fairness. The statements below concern the fairness of fertility decisions and desires with regard to the husband's desires as they are perceived by the wife.

> The last two years were so concentrated that he wasn't thinking about anything except his book, and I think that's why he reacted the way he did when I made the statement that I was going to get a tubal ligation. I realized that wasn't fair on my part, but on the other hand, maybe it was my way of trying to come to a decision.

> He didn't want kids, couldn't see any reason for us to have kids, and I didn't feel it was my right to just get pregnant "by accident." It was something we had to deal with.

The fairness of fertility decisions is considered with regard to people outside the family as well. The childless woman ponders the fairness of her adopting children:

> I wish I could just have a child, without having to go through the pregnancy, which I could if I adopted a child, but then I'd feel really guilty, because there's all these other people who can't have children, and that's not fair to them.

A mother of three recalls her decision to have no more children:

> I really had a strong drive to have another one. I consciously thought that it wouldn't be fair to have more kids. I had three.

Fairness to the child is considered in regard to parental employment choices as this woman who contemplates a career in international development suggests:

> I think it would be very selfish for us to go traipsing off someplace, taking ourselves into consideration more than the little being that's growing inside. I think that's a ridiculous noble savage attitude that people have about what they can do: "Millions of women have had their babies out in the field, so can I."

Women with less exotic career plans also consider fairness in balancing work with responsibility to the child.

> I could not go and work for eight hours, and then try to be civil with my children, even one. It would be difficult. I'd be tired, I have real low blood pressure, and I have a very low metabolism, and I think it would just wear me out. I don't think I could handle it. Maybe I could work half-time. My husband wouldn't care, as long as the baby was happy.

If I had kids, if I was working they would think the same thing I thought about my mother: "There's Mom, why don't I ever do anything with her?" It would be a real loss, somehow. From the kid's point of view I would think that.

Regarding the equality of care children receive:

I want to be able to give my children, all of them, whether it's two or six, the same quality. I don't know whether that's even possible.

I think it is hard to equally love all of your children, but some people are very flagrant about not equally loving their children, and it's caused them some real problems. You have to be careful about trying to be equal, and realize they have different personalities, and what's good for one may not necessarily be good for the other.

Even a woman's assessment of her ability to perform adequately the duties of a mother is couched in terms of fairness:

I really think I felt like I would not be a good parent, and it would not be fair to the child.

To sum up, women use fairness in a wide variety of contexts. Further, in the same way that motivations for childbearing are expressed in terms of nuclear family relationships, the attempt to make fair reproductive decisions tends to focus on nuclear family members and, to a lesser extent, on the wider society.

How this is enacted can be suggested by an example. For one of my informants, the loss of freedom was a major concern for both her and her husband when they conceived their first child. When her husband began to press for another child, her reaction was negative. She felt her freedom would be even more curtailed by a second child and that responsibility for child care fell disproportionately to her. With one child she had felt the need to reduce her job commitment to half-time; with another it would be more difficult to cope, and the children's care would suffer. Having borne a child, she would not deprive her husband of the opportunity to be a father by avoiding a second pregnancy. She felt that all parties, herself, her son, and her husband, were fairly served by her decision to stop at one child.

Conclusions

My conclusions from the interview data are twofold: that fairness, freedom, and responsibility play a major role in women's reasoning about their reproductive decisions, and that the way women apply these principles to their decisions suggests a hierarchy of values. That is, fairness takes precedence over freedom and responsibility, acting as an arbiter when conflicts arise between behaviors that maximize either freedom or responsibility. The rights of the child (prospective or extant) are balanced against the rights of the parents; the rights of the wife against the rights of the husband. Even the rights of extended family members may be considered (in the context of providing grandchildren, for example). Women use all three values to judge if they are having, or not having, children for the proper reasons, and to assess if they have adequately met the emotional and financial prerequisites for parenthood. Used retrospectively, these values provide a rationale for whatever decision is taken.

What of the second objective of this chapter: to clarify the connections between individuals' reproductive decisions and fertility trends in the aggregate? It appears that when women accept and act on the prescription to be fair, independent, and responsible, and apply these principles to their reproductive decisions, fertility tends to be low. Only when fairness is invoked in the cause of providing siblings for existing children can it be said to stimulate fertility. Even so, providing a sibling for the first child requires a total of only two children. Rarely does the propriety of providing siblings extend to providing many siblings. Thus it would appear that cultural and economic phenomena conspire to keep American fertility low for the immediate future. On the other hand, that women call on individualistic principles to shape reproductive decisions may be a source of solace for those who fear continued fertility decline or the policy decisions such fear may prompt. As long as women see childbearing as offering an emotional fulfillment difficult to obtain elsewhere, they may continue to feel that, given the appropriate prerequisites, it is "only fair" to them and their families to have a child. Further, while women may avoid childbearing in the early years of marriage to test the stability of the union, the nearly unbreakable (so our culture would have us believe) bond between mother and child is appealing to women in a land where, by some estimates, half of all marriages end in divorce. These scenarios, played out many times in the population will not ensure a return to high fertility levels, but will impose a floor beneath which fertility will not go.

Finally, what is the significance of these findings for women themselves? Changes in the status of women, especially labor force participation and the economic and personal power so gained, go hand in hand with infusion of the political values associated with individualism into the private sphere of reproductive decisions. This has been facilitated greatly by a contraceptive revolution, including the anovulant birth control pill and the intrauterine device, which has effectively separated the act of intercourse from the attempt to prevent pregnancy. Women in the United States currently make reproductive decisions in a context where the absolute costs of children are high, and the opportunity costs of motherhood continue to increase with education levels and employment opportunities (see Huber 1980). We see high levels of education for women, late age at marriage, massive labor force participation of women, and high incidence of divorce. The principle of fairness provides a balance between the desire to have children and the reluctant perception of the economic realities that make any fertility economically irrational (Caldwell 1976). Not only is fertility "irrational" in economic terms, but other valued roles and activities may have to be foregone if one is to be a mother.

It is clear that reproductive choice can present a dilemma for women. Having children can be hazardous to a woman's career. A woman's full-time job can be detrimental to domestic tranquility. Early aspirations and life course events affect women's paths as they veer toward domesticity or toward career involvement (Gerson 1985). Whichever perspective a woman takes, she faces working a double day if she chooses to have children and work outside the home. Demographic data suggest American women do not feel that choosing *either* motherhood *or* career satisfaction is the answer. As of 1980 nearly 94 percent of ever-married women became mothers by age 44. At the same time, 45 percent of mothers of children under age six and 62 percent of mothers of school age children were in the paid work force (Bianchi and Spain 1983:18).

Under these circumstances, the fact that fairness, freedom, and responsibility are deeply cherished values makes them a perfect vehicle for directing and expressing reproductive decisions. Because individualism is seen as the natural state of human beings, a woman's decisions and actions, taken in the best interests of herself and her family, can be couched in terms acceptable to the wider society, within and outside the family. While the decision may be hard for others to accept (for example, parents may be disappointed when their children do not provide them with grandchildren or that their daughter's education is wasted when she becomes a homemaker), the principle of fairness can hardly be rejected. Rather than being stymied by the choice between freedom and responsibility, women can consider possible alternatives in terms of fairness to the parties involved as a route to resolution.

There is no clear cultural mandate for how modern American women are to make their way in the world. Nearly 25 years after the founding of the National Organization for Women, which may serve as a marker for the beginnings of renewed feminist activism on a national scale, it is difficult to see how far women and men have come, and how well families have adjusted, to the new roles women have been encouraged to fill. Very recently, a "men's movement" has emerged to promote equal consideration for men's domestic roles. A primary focus of their activity is child custody in the event of divorce. That men might feel the need to organize in order to protect their rights from women would have been laughable even 15 years ago. Perhaps this testifies to profound changes in American society. On a more cynical note, it may reflect a backlash against women now that they have gained access to education and economic independence and freedom from compulsory motherhood. In any case, the enduring cultural mandate may be to embrace those principles of individualism which have characterized our culture for so long. It remains to be seen how this course will affect marriage, the family, and the participation of men and women in both the domestic and public spheres and provides fertile grounds for new research.

Acknowledgments

I would like to thank Barbara Entwisle and Penn Handwerker for helpful comments and advice on various drafts of this chapter; the Department of Anthropology of Washington State University where the research was conducted; and the Carolina Population Center which has supported me, as a postdoctoral fellow and visiting scholar, during the preparation of the manuscript. An earlier version of this chapter was presented at the annual meetings of the American Anthropological Association held November 18–22, 1987 in Chicago, Illinois.

References Cited

Bianchi, Suzanne M, and Daphne Spain. 1986. American Women in Transition. Census Monograph Series. New York: Russell Sage Foundation.

———. 1983. U.S. Bureau of the Census, Special Demographic Analyses. CDS-80-8. American Women: Three Decades of Change. Washington D.C. U.S. Government Printing Office.

Bulatao, R. A. 1981. Values and Disvalues of Children in Successive Childbearing Decisions. Demography. 11:25–44.

Caldwell, John C. 1976. Toward a Restatement of Demographic Transition Theory. Population and Development Review. 2:321–366.

Cooper, Pamela E., Barbara Cumber, and Robin Hartner. 1978. Decision-making Patterns and Post-decision Adjustment of Childfree Husbands and Wives. Alternate Lifestyles. 1:71–94.

Degler, Carl N. 1980. At Odds: Women and the Family in America from the Revolution to the Present. New York: Oxford University Press.

Fawcett, James T. 1978. The Value and Cost of a Child. In The First Child and Family Formation. Warren B. Miller and Lucille F. Newman, editors. Pp.

244–265. Chapel Hill, North Carolina: Carolina Population Center, The University of North Carolina at Chapel Hill.

Gabriel, Ayala. 1983. Male/Female Models of Motivation for Reproduction among Dual Occupation Couples. Paper presented at the 82nd Annual Meetings of the American Anthropological Association.

Gerson, Kathleen. 1985. Hard Choices: How Women Decide about Work, Career, and Motherhood. Berkeley, California: University of California Press.

Hochschild, Jennifer L. 1981. What's Fair?: American Beliefs about Distributive Justice. Cambridge, Massachusetts, and London, England: Harvard University Press.

Hsu, Francis L. K. 1972. American Core Value and National Character. *In* Psychological Anthropology. Francis L. K. Hsu, editor. Pp. 209–230. Cambridge, Massachusetts: Schenkman Publishers.

Huber, Joan. 1980. Will U.S. Fertility Decline Toward Zero? The Sociological Quarterly. 21:481–492.

Leone, Catherine L. 1986. Fairness, Freedom, and Responsibility: The Dilemma of Fertility Choice in America. Ph.D. dissertation. Department of Anthropology. Washington State University. Pullman, Washington.

Macfarlane, Alan. 1978. The Origins of English Individualism: Some Surprises. Theory and Society 6:255–277.

8

The Politics of Choice:
Abortion as Insurrection

Warren M. Hern

News Item: Joseph Scheidler, founder of the Chicago-based Pro-Life Action League, claimed victory after staging a two-hour picket in front of the Boulder Abortion Clinic yesterday morning. Because no women came in for abortions during that time, Scheidler said he had shut the clinic down for the morning. Dr. Warren Hern, who performs the clinic's abortions, denied that appointments were changed in anticipation of the picket. But Scheidler . . . insisted that no clients showed up "because I'm here."

—Colorado Daily, Wednesday, October 23, 1985

A Personal Prologue

I have worked in some aspect of fertility control for twenty years. I have spent more than fifteen of those years providing abortion services, but the last three years have been among the most memorable in my experience. On October 18, 1985, a large stone was thrown through the front window of my office by an antiabortion supporter of Joseph Scheidler, who was due to arrive in Boulder that weekend (Langer, 1985). Mr. Scheidler spent a considerable part of his time in Colorado attacking me and inciting others to do so as well. His favorite place for mounting this attack was the sidewalk in front of my office (Brennan, 1985a,b; Roberts 1985; Putnam 1985; Bortnick 1985; Gelchion 1985). There, he encountered a phalanx of eight Boulder policemen, two private security guards, and two representatives of the Boulder District Attorney's office. In spite of his promises to risk arrest by trying to take over my office, he backed down and left for Chicago claiming he had "closed" my office. Scheidler claims to have "closed" 34 clinics.

In the week following Scheidler's first ignominious visit to Boulder, Colorado, I received a half-dozen death threats. My clinic had a bomb

127

threat. We had hundreds of hang-up calls in attempts to jam the telephones. Picketers became more aggressive.

In early December, Scheidler returned to demonstrate at my office again and to hold more rallies. The number of hostile calls increased, and aggressive picketing resumed following his departure. Scheidler threatened to return again on December 28, the "Day of Rescue," but he didn't. Instead, we were hounded by dozens of phony service calls and deliveries (Brennan, 1986a). We began receiving large quantities of unsolicited junk mail, books, and subscriptions. I criticized the Colorado Right to Life Committee and one of its leaders, and they sued me for slander and asked for $2 million dollars (Horsley 1986; Brennan 1986b).

Mr. Scheidler's next appearance was at Orlando, Florida. There, according to eyewitness reports, he rolled up to an abortion clinic in a Cadillac Eldorado and was whisked away by private jet after his demonstration.

The Orlando clinic that Scheidler visited has been the target of Scheidler and his fanatic followers since at least July, 1983. The clinic was sprayed with gunfire in January, 1984. The clinic director has received numerous death threats (personal communication, clinic director).

Bombs and Bullets Are Not Theoretical

In 1987, the Alan Guttmacher Institute (AGI) published the results of a survey of the harassment of U.S. abortion service providers. Of the 400 non-hospital abortion providers, 88 percent had experienced antiabortion harassment in 1985, 29 percent had been invaded and vandalized, and 20 percent had had their phones jammed by phony calls. Fifty-two percent had been forced to increase security costs, 32 percent had lost malpractice insurance, and 24 percent had lost fire and casualty insurance. Seventy-three percent of the clinics were targets of illegal activities (Forrest, 1987). "In no other U.S. setting," say the AGI authors, "are health care workers likely to be threatened for providing services that are legal."

In my own survey of 150 National Abortion Federation member clinics, 29 percent had experienced serious violence, including total destruction of facilities, sometimes more than once; 26 percent had been visited by Scheidler; 45 percent had experienced increasingly aggressive harassment, frequently associated with Scheidler's visits; 35 percent had lost insurance coverage; and 26 percent had received death threats, bomb threats, or both.

A live bomb was delivered to a Portland, Oregon clinic in December, 1985, and three others were found in the Portland postal system the same day (Clendinen, 1985). One was addressed to a physician who performs abortions and who had been the target of death threats and two arson attempts. The bombs were designed to kill whoever opened the package.

At a national conference of radical antiabortion activists in Appleton, Wisconsin held in the summer of 1985, participants wore buttons saying, "Have a Blast."

President Reagan and his advisers have said that there is no national conspiracy and no terrorism against abortion clinics (Washington Times, 1987). From 1977 until 1981, there were 69 aggressive or violent incidents against abortion clinics. Thirteen included bombing or arson, and two of the arsons resulted in total destruction of the facility. Since Ronald Reagan took office in 1981, there have been 778 violent or aggressive incidents against abortion clinics, of which 57 have included bombing or arson, and facilities were completely destroyed in fourteen cases (National Abortion Federation, 1988).

On November 20, 1987, antiabortion propagandist Bernard Nathanson stated at a press conference and in a speech in Denver that antiabortion pressure is building and would have to be released or "there will be violence" (Rocky Mountain News, 21 November 1987). Nathanson made a point of attacking me in his remarks.

On January 25, 1988, Reagan attacked abortion in his State of the Union message before Congress (New York Times, 26 January 1988). A few days later, on January 30, the Reagan administration issued new regulations forbidding personnel at federally-funded family planning clinics from even mentioning abortion to patients (Pear, 1988). On February 2, the Planned Parenthood Federation and several clinics including some in Colorado filed suit to enjoin the regulations (Lewin, 1988).

The next day, February 3, Republican Presidential candidate Pat Robertson made a highly inflammatory speech against abortion before the New Hampshire state legislature and stated that Planned Parenthood was trying to develop a "master race" (Dees, 1988).

On February 4, 1988, five shots were fired into the front of my office building (Daily Camera, 5 February 1988; Robey 1988; Black 1988). Three bullets passed through the glass into the waiting room. I had just left the area, and an employee working in the building narrowly escaped injury.

No matter what the Supreme Court says, I find it necessary from time to time to work under the protection of armed private security guards to protect my patients and staff. We have installed bullet-proof windows and electronic protective devices in my clinic.

The harassment continues across the nation. On May 2, 1988, 500 people belonging to an organization called "Operation Rescue" demonstrated against a New York abortion clinic (Brozan 1988). Nearly 600 demonstrators were arrested at a Paoli, Pennsylvania abortion clinic on 5 July, and 250 demonstrated at a nearby clinic the next day (Mayer 1988; Enda 1988a,b). On June 19, 1988, a series of aggressive demonstrations led by Rev. Jerry Falwell began in Atlanta and continued for weeks (Smothers 1988).

These events underscore the nature of the current struggle to maintain freedom of reproductive choice in America today. That struggle is being waged on many fronts. Many important battles have been lost, at least for now. We have won some important victories, especially in the courts. Scheidler and his goons represent the effort to drive abortion services underground and to reduce them to essentially the same status as prevailed in the days when abortion was illegal. The tactics are ruthless and insidious; they include telephone harassment and obstruction of clinic telephone lines, false and misleading advertisement of the so-called "pregnancy crisis" clinics, picketing of not only clinics but doctors' homes and churches, telephone harassment and picketing of other clinic personnel, harassment of patients and invasion of privacy, disruption of pro-choice meetings, clinic invasions, covert actions, death threats, and numerous other iniquitous methods. Many of these tactics are described in Scheidler's book, *Closed: 99 Ways to Stop Abortion* (Scheidler 1985).

Mr. Scheidler claims he does not condone violence. Yet he praises and "sympathizes" with those who commit violence against abortion clinics, and he visits them in jail. He states he will not condemn violence, and stated in Colorado that violence has a place in his movement (Putnam, 1985). He is fond of stating, "I have yet to shed my first tear over the smoldering remains of an abortion clinic" (Donovan 1985).

Many of those who find abortion abhorrent and even some who work actively to outlaw it find Scheidler's tactics unacceptable. He has been thrown out of the mainstream Right-To-Life Committee organization at several levels (Cancila 1985). But he accurately symbolizes and represents an important segment of antiabortion radicals who will literally stop at nothing to disrupt abortion services.

For those of us who provide services, this strategy produces nightmarish problems. It threatens basic personal freedoms. The rhetoric of violence employed by Scheidler and others like him chills our participation in community life and endangers our lives. We are highly vulnerable to these attacks.

To us, the antiabortion fanatics are those we must face daily, not our reasonable friends and colleagues with whom we can courteously disagree and with whom we maintain not only professional relationships but friendships. We do not see or hear so much from those who sincerely disagree with abortion but who reject the methods of Scheidler and Falwell.

The courts have agreed that we have the right to provide contraceptive and abortion services, but we struggle in reality each day to maintain those rights against the scurrilous tactics of people like Scheidler and those who support him. We have not yet won the political battle for reproductive freedom, much less abortion, in this country.

Changes in American social attitudes toward abortion during the past 150 years have crystallized during the past 5 years into a pitched battle between abortion service providers and those who are determined to prevent abortions from being performed. This is not merely a battle in the abstract sense; bombs and bullets are not theoretical.

Antiabortion National Politics

President Reagan is the first American president to make opposition to abortion a prime tenet of his political program, and he is the first to invoke both official and unofficial strategies to accomplish his goal. At his first press conference on the day after he was elected in November, 1980, he announced one of his primary goals as outlawing abortion (Kneeland 1980). On his inauguration day in January, 1981, he met with leaders of antiabortion groups. Reagan's new Secretary of Health and Human Services, Richard Schweiker, spoke that day to an antiabortion rally and promised the group a "pro-life" administration (UPI, 1981).

Abortion and the Conscience of the Nation, an antiabortion tract purportedly written by Reagan, appeared in 1984 (Reagan 1984). It included an antiabortion speech by Dr. C. Everett Koop, who had just been appointed Surgeon General of the United States by Reagan. The speech was entitled, "The Slide To Auschwitz." Reagan was the first President to recognize and address the annual March for Life in Washington, D.C. On January 22, 1985, he told the rally, "I feel a great sense of solidarity with all of you" (Clendinen 1985b). Each year during his presidency, on January 22, Reagan honored antiabortion leaders by meeting them personally in the White House. In 1986, he was asked by those leaders to pardon the abortion clinic bombers (Brown 1986), and he never issued a clear repudiation of the suggestion. One of those with whom Reagan regularly met, and who participated in the appeal to pardon abortion clinic bombers, is Joseph Scheidler.

In January, 1985, following a series of particularly destructive abortion clinic bombings, one of which occurred in Washington, D.C. (Associate Press, New York Times, 1984; Hershey 1985), Reagan issued a brief press release condemning the bombings (Boyd 1985). Reagan's only other statement indicating concern for the violence directed toward women and doctors and others who help them in abortion clinics was delivered as an amplified message to an antiabortion rally at the Ellipse in January, 1987.

The Republican Party has adopted three successive national platforms with clear statements of opposition both to equal rights for women and to reproductive freedom. At the National Right To Life Convention held in Denver in June, 1986, three prospective Republican presidential candidates, Bob Dole, Pat Robertson, and Jack Kemp, were featured as speakers (Obmascik 1986). George Bush was on the program but begged off. The Republicans know where to find the votes; the antiabortion activists know where to find the power.

The antipathy toward abortion goes far beyond any particular individual's moral outrage or philosophic difference. Almost more than any other social movement in the twentieth century, the antiabortion movement has sought—and gained—political power with the objective of restricting freedom. In this respect, it is clearly distinguished from the civil rights movement of the 60s, which sought to enlarge freedom for a class of people whose rights under the Constitution were clearly established but effectively and systematically denied.

The drive for political power by antiabortion groups, and the drive to impose a specific view of women and to restrict women's rights, suggests that some previous occurrence in political history compelled this reaction. The provocative event, or series of events, is not hard to identify.

From the early part of the twentieth century, concentrated efforts have been made to provide effective means of fertility control both to men and to women (Peel and Potts 1969; Himes 1970). The 1965 Griswold v. Connecticut and the 1973 Roe v. Wade and Doe v. Bolton decisions completed an historic progression in the establishment of safe fertility control as a right for women.

We who have been providing abortion services since 1973 have seen implementation of the 1973 decision as the greatest challenge of our lives. Hostility toward abortion service providers has waxed and waned since 1973; it is now on the rise and it is increasingly vicious toward patients, doctors, and other health personnel. In 1973, it took the form of personal insults and attacks on our competence and character in hospital staff meetings, attempts to keep us from obtaining hospital privileges, and attempts to pass resolutions against us in the medical society meetings.

Since the election of President Reagan in 1980, things have become worse. We feel this hostility and the pressure in our everyday lives, even when we are not being directly assaulted. At this point, we do not feel protected by the Supreme Court decisions.

The court decisions were made possible by advances in medical technology, especially in contraceptive technology. Safe and effective fertility control, in general, especially abortion, permits radical new views of pregnancy, childbearing, marriage, and the role of women.

But Why Abortion?

The question remains: why is abortion such a focus for conflict in this massive change in the role of women and increased safety for women? Why does morbid fascination with the fetus become such an emotional pivot point?

Why is abortion such a controversial issue in our society? More to the point for me personally, why would I want to be involved in the issue? How did I become involved? Why, in fact, do I remain involved? Is it possible now for me not to be involved?

The abortion controversy exists not because of those who have abortions or those who perform them. It exists because of the intense feelings of those who are bystanders and who are not affected directly by the act of abortion. Why, then are they who oppose abortion so intently determined to prevent others from acting?

Some Public Health History

To answer these questions, we must begin with the fact that human beings have limited their fertility in some form or another throughout human existence (Himes 1970). Anthropologists think, for example, that the human population grew at the rate of 0.001 percent per year for hundreds of thousands of years (Hassan 1981). At least part of the reason for that slow growth had to be the result of limitations on fertility, although it is hard to tell how much of the limitation was conscious. We know that conscious efforts to limit fertility occurred in the ancient societies of the Mediterranean and Middle East, including Egypt (Himes 1970:59-202). We know that small-scale societies throughout the world have methods to limit family size (Nag 1976; Hern 1976). These include genital mutilation, folk systems of limiting intercourse in sexual contact, ritual sexual abstinence, postpartum sexual abstinence, abortion, and infanticide.

Anthropologist George Devereaux described the practice of abortion in some 300 traditional societies around the world (Devereux 1955). Before Christian missionaries set them straight, Tikopians limited fertility by some of these means because they recognized that their small Pacific island would not sustain unlimited growth of the human population (Firth 1957). Thanks to the missionaries, their demographic control mechanisms were disrupted and the Tikopia found themselves uncomfortably crowded on their island.

In English Common Law, abortion was considered a misdemeanor unless it occurred after "quickening," when the woman could feel movement of the fetus (Means 1968, 1971). It was only in the 19th century that American legislatures began to pass laws against abortion. Part of the reason for the laws was that abortion, at that time, was considered more dangerous than carrying the pregnancy to term (Roe v. Wade, 410 U.S. 113, 149 (1973)). Margaret Sanger saw that women were dying from illegal and unsafe abortions, and this was a powerful impetus for her campaign for contraception. Today, legal abortion not only saves the lives of women but increases the chance that women who are poor or are members of minority groups will survive pregnancy (Gold 1965).

Could it be that that fact has something to do with the opposition to abortion in our society?

In old obstetrics textbooks, and even some new ones, one finds statements to the effect that "pregnancy is the most normal thing that can happen to a woman" or "a woman is most 'normal' when she is pregnant." Pregnancy is "the highest function of the female reproductive system and a priori should be considered a normal process" (Eastman and Hellman 1961). At one conference, an obstetrician defined a woman as a "uterus surrounded by a supporting organism and a directing personality" (Calderone 1958). At another conference, a woman psychoanalyst stated that "any woman who has conflicts about being pregnant or wants to have an abortion" is by definition psychopathological (Romm 1967). She is sick. It is not surprising that the early 1960s saw the phenomenon of requiring women who sought abortions to see psychiatrists who would declare them mentally ill so that abortions could be obtained. Mental illness, of course, could be the only justification for abortion since the pregnancy was "normal" and the woman was "healthy." This arrangement did, of course, require that women negotiate the power structure of medical authority in order to obtain relief from an unwanted pregnancy that threatened to disrupt her life.

Is Pregnancy Normal?

Is pregnancy "normal"? Is it "normal" for a woman to be pregnant? It is common, to be sure. It is a lot more common among some groups and in certain parts of the world than in others, but does that make it "normal"? In parts of Switzerland and in parts of Latin America, nearly everyone has a goiter as the result of iodine deficiencies in the local diet. In these places, it has been considered "normal" to have a goiter. But is it "normal" (Hern 1971)?

It is common for a Shipibo Indian woman in the upper Amazon Basin of Peru to be pregnant for a total of 45 percent of the time during her reproductive years (Hern 1977). It is likely that a white woman living in Boulder, Colorado or Des Moines, Iowa will be pregnant for only 5 percent of the time during her reproductive years. For which woman is pregnancy "normal"?

In fact, both women have a risk of dying of pregnancy, although the risks are different. If a woman has a certifiable, definable, and measurable risk of dying as the result of pregnancy, how can pregnancy be "normal"? If a woman is in her "normal" state when she is pregnant, what is she when she is not pregnant? Obviously, if her personhood and meaning in existence depends on her being pregnant and reproducing, she can only be "normal" when she is pregnant. That definition of women, as it happens, suits some people very well. For one thing, it helps maintain a male power structure by keeping women occupied with reproduction.

In a 1963 speech before the Little Rock Optimist Club, the late Arkansas legislator Paul Van Dalsem said, "I'll tell you what we do up in Perry County when one of our women starts poking around in something she doesn't know anything about. We get her an extra milk cow. If that don't work, we get her a little more garden to tend, and if that's not enough, we get her pregnant and keep her barefoot" (Reed 1963).

Van Dalsem had cause for concern about women meddling in important matters. In the next election, women who called themselves "Barefoot Women For Rule" campaigned barefoot and in sunbonnets for Herbert Rule, Van Dalsem's opponent. Van Dalsem lost the election. Arkansas women now bestow an annual "Uppity Woman" award to commemorate this political event.

More recently, 1988 Republican Presidential aspirant Pat Robertson, the TV evangelist, expressed his concerns that we will not have enough taxpayers to pay the bills and, by implication, soldiers to fight wars if the availability of abortion reduces the number of children that women bear (King 1987).

The idea that pregnancy is "normal" and that it is the highest objective for women's lives has important political consequences, especially for those who see women primarily as reproductive machines to serve the power of the state and those who control it. As a scientist and physician, however, I am interested in looking at views of pregnancy as hypotheses and testing their validity as hypotheses. The usefulness of any hypothesis depends on its ability to explain reality and predict events. The hypothesis that pregnancy is "normal," unfortunately, does not explain anything we know about pregnancy and does not predict any events related to pregnancy. It does not explain the fact, for example, that there is a

specific etiology of pregnancy, that physiologic changes occur in women
when they are pregnant, that these changes may be documented by
laboratory studies, that the changes lead to a risk of death that is
increased over the nonpregnant state, that the death rate due to pregnancy
(a.k.a. "maternal mortality rate") is a well-documented phenomenon,
that pregnancy is a self-limiting condition from which spontaneous
recovery usually, but not always, occurs, that we may modify the risk
of death due to pregnancy by certain cultural innovations (e.g. medical
intervention), that the susceptibility to pregnancy varies by sex and
other factors, that the condition of pregnancy is universally but unevenly
distributed among the human species, that pregnancy is preventable, as
are other illness conditions, and that human beings throughout the world
display "illness behavior," "sick role behavior," and "health behavior"
with regard to pregnancy.

The hypothesis that pregnancy is "normal" does not explain any of
these observations, and it does not predict any of them.

Pregnancy as Illness

This being the case, what is an alternative hypothesis? An alternative
hypothesis is that pregnancy is an illness (Hern 1975). It has a specific
etiology, pathogenesis, pathophysiology, laboratory findings, clinical manifestations, signs, symptoms, duration, prevalence, incidence, susceptibility, distribution pattern, and case fatality rate. It may be diagnosed
by various means, its course may be influenced by medical or surgical
management, it may be prevented, and screening techniques may be
employed to determine the community incidence and prevalence.

If pregnancy is an illness, however, how is it that we are all here?
Why didn't we all die out thousands of years ago? One answer is that
pregnancy is a biological adaptation to the survival needs of the species.
Like other biological adaptations, it may have certain survival advantages
for the species and certain disadvantages for individual members of the
species.

Sickle cell trait is another example. Heterozygous inheritance of the
sickle cell trait in West Africa protects against falciparum malaria
(Medawar 1960). It is a biological adaptation that has helped the species
survive in West Africa. Homozygous inheritance leads to sickle cell
disease, a painful and incurable condition leading to early death in the
small proportion of individuals who experience it. Those individuals die
as the result of an adaptation that protects many others.

In 1920, the maternal mortality rate in the United States was 680
per 100,000 live births (Lerner and Anderson 1963:34). In 1960, it was
about 30 (1963:32). It is now down to about 14 (Rochat et al. 1988),

but it is not zero, and it probably never will be. It has been reduced principally because of the introduction of modern obstetrical practices including medical management of high-risk pregnancies, the introduction of modern surgical techniques including asepsis, anesthesia, and blood transfusions, and the introduction of modern antibiotics. It has also been reduced by the introduction of modern contraceptives that permit delays in the occurrence of first pregnancy, longer birth intervals, and fewer total pregnancies per woman.

The availability of safe legal abortion has also been instrumental in reducing maternal mortality rates. Dr. Christopher Tietze estimated in 1984 that at least 1500 women had not died in the United States since 1970 as the result of the legalization of abortion (Tietze 1984).

If pregnancy were really normal, we wouldn't have worried about doing any of those things, and they wouldn't have made much difference.

If pregnancy is an illness, why do we persist in calling it "normal" and hauling out the party hats when some unfortunate woman has quintuplets?

Calling pregnancy "normal" and celebrating fecundity, even extraordinary fecundity, is a cultural adaptation to the survival needs of our species. These values were adaptive when we were a few thousand struggling bands of nomadic hunters and gatherers scattered about the globe. They were possibly even adaptive at the end of the 14th century when the Black Death had wiped out as much as one-third of the human population from India to Iceland (Tuchman 1978). As the human population passes the 5 billion mark and every day brings new reports of ominous and even permanent destruction of the global environment, from deforestation of Madagascar to collapse of the Peruvian anchovy schools to desertification and famine in Africa to disappearance of the ozone layer in the Antarctic to death of the Mediterranean and Baltic Seas to accelerating destruction of the Amazon rain forest, when we find that the human population is no longer increasing at the rate of 0.001 percent per year or 0.1 percent per year but 2, 3, and 4 percent per year in particular locations, when we are destroying natural habitats and extinguishing other species at a rate too rapid to be measured, and when the major cities of the world are becoming uninhabitable from crowding and congestion, we must consider the possibility that the view that human pregnancy is "normal" or even glorious is no longer adaptive. In fact, it very well might be maladaptive. It might reduce our capacity to survive as a species. We already know it is maladaptive for individual women in countries like the United States.

We may even go so far as to say that abortion is the treatment of choice for pregnancy unless the woman clearly wishes to carry the pregnancy to term and to reproduce. Even then, the risks to her and to the planet must be taken seriously

Political Implications of Abortion

It is by no means necessary to accept the idea of pregnancy as an "illness" in order to support the need for fertility control, including abortion, for individuals and for the species. Having recognized the fact that the prevention of pregnancy and availability of treatment of pregnancy by abortion is desirable both from the woman's point of view and from the point of a rational human society, however, what are we to make of the intense opposition to abortion not to mention opposition to fertility control in general by some groups in our society?

The most fervent antiabortion groups are led and directed by men (Luker 1984); Scheidler is the most lurid example. These men tend to espouse a regressive if not totalitarian philosophy that requires subservience for women and control of social institutions by men (Merton, 1981). Here is Scheidler in a 1984 interview with American Medical News, while expressing his opposition to the Equal Rights Amendment: "It would give women the same rights as men. . . . God didn't intend that or he wouldn't have had women bearing children" (Cancila 1985).

Scheidler's statement exposes the real objectives of the antiabortion movement. Opposition to reproductive freedom in general and to abortion in particular appears to reflect profound antipathy toward the changing roles of women in our society.

Antiabortion groups represent a cultural counterrevolution that resists and tries to repeal profound changes that have occurred in our society in the last century, particularly during the past 30 years. The introduction of safe and effective fertility control measures in the last quarter-century has freed women to choose not to reproduce and to choose to develop other skills in society. Women have new opportunities for education and for careers.

Abortion is the most obvious, vulnerable, and dramatic example of the new freedom for women. It is the final and irretrievable act of fertility control a woman can exercise in a particular pregnancy. Abortion is therefore truly revolutionary in the sense that it fundamentally and irreversibly changes power relations within Western society. It is an ultimate act of insurrection against male control of womens' lives.

Kristin Luker has shown that antiabortion and pro-choice women activists have radically different world views (1984). Those opposed to abortion are likely to see reproduction and motherhood as not only a primary role but a moral obligation for women. However they may see pregnancy as a condition, pro-choice activists studied by Luker tend to see reproduction as one of the options in life, along with other meaningful activities.

To the historic patriarchal agrarian society and those who defend its values, abortion is an act of insurrection. It shatters the last bonds of biological tyranny that have been used to control the lives of women and some men. Women, freed from the tyranny of biology, have become uppity. They now compete with men for jobs, money, and power. The effort to crush those who provide this service and to crush all progress toward equality for women in our society raises fundamental questions.

Those who defend the traditional values say that the problem is the definition of human life and that our definition is inadequate.

The issue, however, is not when life begins, but who is best prepared to make the decision to transmit life to a new generation: the individual or the state?

The issue is not the definition of life but the definition of power: who has it, and who doesn't. Will power in our society be wielded absolutely by those who cannot become pregnant, or will it be shared by those who can?

The fetus becomes a pawn in this power struggle. It becomes a demigod, a fetish object to be protected against evil. It is endowed with magical and fantastic properties, as we see in the propaganda movie, "The Silent Scream." Fetus fetish dolls even become a source of revenue for the Right to Life movement (National Right to Life News, October 24, 1986, p. 7).

Fetuses are politically useful. They are not uppity and they do not argue. They present no economic threat to the male power structure. They can be defended along with the flag and motherhood before the voters at election time. They can be defended against sin and immorality, thereby throwing political opponents into disarray. It is an irresistible opportunity for the exercise of righteous indignation.

The reason why opposition to abortion works so well as a political organizing issue is that it plays well both to the emotions of simple people who wish to defend traditional values and to righteous fanatics who see themselves as the defenders of public virtue. It supports the activities of those who feel good by making other people feel bad. It supports those who fear thought, reason, intellectual and academic freedom, and those who fear the participation in democratic society of those who are different.

Defending the fetus also is an effective way to divert attention away from other intractable and less interesting matters of public policy such as the national debt, staggering budget deficits, the arms race, colossal environmental destruction, uncontrolled growth of the human population, poverty and malnutrition, illiteracy, and epidemic disease subsidized by the tobacco industry. Opposition to abortion thus becomes a path to political power, as the Reagan and Bush regimes so clearly demonstrate.

Under the Reagan administration, abortion became an overt political act. As Reagan, Bush, and their henchmen move to crush the insurrection, abortion is in danger of becoming a political crime against the state.

Scheidler and Falwell are merely henchmen for the right wing's war on women and basic personal freedoms. Scheidler, Falwell, and others like them want power, and fanatic opposition to abortion is a tool for obtaining power. Their methods and contempt for the rights of others link them with all the tyrants of history. That their friends in the White House seem to be such nice guys does not diminish the cruelty and danger of this threat to liberty. That a man like Scheidler must travel all the way from Chicago to Boulder, Colorado or to Orlando, Florida to try to stop us from what we are doing must mean we are doing something important to advance the cause of human freedom.

Abortion has become a political issue because it is about power. It is about who runs your life. It is about who runs our society. It is about self-determination, about self-realization, about individual choice, about personal freedom and responsibility. It is about humanistic values as distinguished from supernatural, fantastic, or divine control of human lives as interpreted by those who claim that they speak with God and Authority.

Opposition to legal abortion, in the long run, is an exercise in futility, notwithstanding temporary successes in restricting access to abortion and the vexation of mindless harassment. As social scientists, we might understand that there is a cultural lag between the fundamentalist prayer meeting message that harshly condemns abortion for "moral" reasons and the currents of late 20th century urban society. As citizens, though, we must perceive the threat to civil liberties and modern political order and consider our responses.

Some Personal Conclusions

I must ask myself what my own role is in this process. Does it matter that I perform abortions? Does it matter that I defend the right of physicians to do so? Does it matter that I defend the right of women not only to have them, but to have them under conditions of safe, humane, supportive medical care?

This is not an abstract issue. In this case, words do not fulfill the freedom to choose. After someone decides to have an abortion, someone must be ready to perform it. For some people, I am half of that equation.Abortion is not the best answer to every unplanned or unwanted pregnancy, and it is not the answer to every complicated pregnancy. It requires a difficult and sometimes extremely painful personal decision, it carries some physical risk, especially if not performed properly, and it is often physically painful. It is for many a cause of great sadness, especially when it occurs without adequate psychological support under degrading or dangerous conditions. Under safe and humane conditions, it can be a source of great relief and an opportunity to begin life anew. But it is never easy for either women who have abortions or for those who provide them (Hern and Corrigan 1979).

My participation in the provision of abortion services as it has occurred in my life could be seen in various ways. To a considerable extent, however, it is the direct consequence of my own logic, conclusions, and personal ethics. I chose medicine because it appeared to be an interesting career with unlimited opportunities for personal service to humanity, opportunities for scientific learning and research, opportunities to relieve suffering, and opportunities for personal growth. I have always been concerned with broad issues of public health. As I worked in some of those issues and saw the connection between individual suffering and public health issues, I kept noticing that women were suffering and dying unnecessarily from illegal abortion. I also observed that failure to provide opportunities for fertility control might unnecessarily increase the rate at which the human population grew and exacerbate the destruction of the very resources needed to sustain it.

Having accepted an invitation to provide abortion services for what I expected to be a relatively short time, I found myself at the center of a controversy far more significant than my own personal choices. I also found that what I did appeared to make important differences in the lives of the women I helped and in the lives of their families. It is very difficult to walk away from circumstances like that.

Now I find myself, some fifteen years later, seeing that I have spent a good part of my life engaged in this struggle. There is no end to the struggle in sight. Shall I continue? Does it matter? Will not others continue the struggle as well if not better? What about my own desire to remove myself from the maelstrom of controversy that threatens my patients, disrupts my life, indeed, threatens at times to interrupt my life?

One ineluctable fact is that before a pregnant woman decides to walk into my office for her appointment with me to have an abortion, the probability is overwhelming that she will have a baby. Her life would be changed. The world would have a new person. In some remote and infinitesimal way, perhaps impossible to measure, we would all be affected. Even so, no decisions are more personal or the result of individual will than the decisions to have sexual intercourse, to have a child, or to have an abortion.

When that woman walks out of my office, she will not be having a baby, at least as the result of that pregnancy. Her life has been changed. Biology is not her destiny, to contradict Freud. We have turned the history of the species upside down. We have changed history. We have changed the world and the relationship of that woman to the world. The fact that we can do this for many women changes our society. The fact that others oppose our actions and would seek to impose the coercive power of the state, to imprison us for our actions, is a political fact that we have, acting together, defied. We have stated that human beings are responsible for their actions, are responsible for the problems created by those actions, and are responsible for the solutions. We have stated that we may change the future, that we may make the world better, that we may choose not to accept the authority of those who would rule by force, ignorance, and fear, and that we may apply human learning and reason to human problems. We have stated that destiny is what we make it, and in a way, that the idea of destiny is no longer valid. We create our lives as we go.

Each one of us who performs abortions, at least those who do so openly, provide a symbolic expression of that idea. As a symbol, it communicates an unfettered message to everyone in our society. The longer that symbol exists, the longer it survives attack, the more it connects with the real needs of real people, the more validity it acquires. That is why the attacks are so direct and increasingly harsh.

As long as that expression of freedom, reason, human caring, and enlargement of human choice is threatened by a totalitarian and oppressive movement, I will perform abortions.

References Cited

Associated Press. 1984. Abortion Clinic and 2 Doctor's offices in Pensacola, Fla, Bombed. New York Times, 26 December.

Black, K. 1988. Shots fired at abortion clinic; director to beef up security. Colorado Daily, 8 February.

Bondeson, W.B., et al. (eds). 1983. Abortion and the Status of the Fetus. Dordrecht, D. Reidel Publishing Company.

Bortnick, B. 1985. Abortion foe greeted by jeers. Daily Times Call, 22 October.

Boyd, G.M. 1985. Reagan condemns arson at clinics. New York Times, 4 January. p. 1.

Brennan, C. 1985a. Anti-abortion leader targets Boulder clinic. Rocky Mountain News, 22 October.

――――. 1985b. Abortion foe skips confrontation. Rocky Mountain News, 23 October.

――――. 1986a. Abortion clinic falls victim of phony service calls. Rocky Mountain News, 3 January.

————. 1986b. Abortionist sued by foes for $2 million. Rocky Mountain News, 18 January.

Brown, P. 1986. Reagan tells abortion foes he's with 'em. Rocky Mountain News, 23 January.

Brozan, N. 1988. 503 protesting abortions are arrested in Manhattan. New York Times, 3 May. p. 14.

Calderone, M. (ed). 1958. Abortion in the United States. New York: Harper-Hoeber.

Cancila, C. 1985. Insider describes anti-MD tactics. American Medical News, 25 January. p. 3.

Clendinen, D. 1985a. Abortion clinics are targets again. New York Times, 9 December, p. B9.

————. 1985b. President praises foes of abortion. New York Times, 23 January. p. 1.

Dees, L. 1988. Pro-Life Pressure: Abortion bill draws hundreds. Concord Monitor, 3 February. p. B1.

Daily Camera. 1988. Shots shatter front window of Boulder Abortion Clinic. Daily Camera, 5 February.

Devereux, G. 1955. A Study of Abortion in Primitive Societies. New York: Julian Press.

Donovan, P. 1985. The Holy War. Family Planning Perspectives 17:5–9.

Eastman, N.J. and L.M. Hellman. 1961. Williams' Obstetrics, 12th ed. New York: Appleton-Century-Crofts.

Enda, J. 1988a. Nearly 600 people arrested in Paoli at abortion clinic. The Philadelphia Inquirer, 6 July.

————. 1988b. Abortion foes block a 2nd clinic. The Philadelphia Inquirer, 7 July.

Firth, R. 1957. We the Tikopia. Boston: Beacon Press.

Forrest, J.D. and S.K. Henshaw. 1987. The Harassment of U.S. Abortion Providers. Family Planning Perspectives 19:9–13.

Gelchion, R. 1985. Doctor, activist trade verbal blows. Daily Times Call, 22 October.

Gold, E.M., et al. 1965. Therapeutic Abortions in New York City: A 20 Year Review. American Journal of Public Health 55:964–972.

Hassan, F. 1981. Demographic Archeology. New York: Academic Press.

Hern, W.M. 1971. Is Pregnancy Really Normal? Family Planning Perspectives 3:5–10.

————. 1975. The Illness Parameters of Pregnancy. Social Science and Medicine 9:365–372.

————. 1976. Knowledge and Use of Herbal Contraceptives in a Peruvian Amazon Village. Human Organization 35:9–19.

————. 1977. High Fertility in a Peruvian Amazon Indian Village. Human Ecology 5:355–368.

Hern, W.M. and B. Corrigan. 1980. What About Us? Staff Reactions to D & C Abortion. Advances in Planning Parenthood 15:3–8.

Hershey, R.D., Jr. 1985. Abortion center in capital bombed. New York Times, 2 January.

Himes, N.E. 1970. Medical History of Contraception. New York: Schocken Books.

Horsley, L. 1986. Abortion opponent sues Hern. Daily Camera, 18 January.

King, W. 1987. Robertson urges policy to increase birth rate. New York Times, 24 October. p. 9.

Kneeland, D.E. 1980. Triumphant Reagan starting transition to the White House. New York Times, 7 November. pp. A1, A14.

Langer, B. 1985. Man throws brick through window of abortion clinic. Daily Camera, 19 October.

Lerner, M. and O.W. Anderson. 1963. Health Progress in the United States: 1900-1960. Chicago: University of Chicago Press.

Lewin, T. 1988. Groups challenge rules on what clinics may say about abortion. New York Times, 2 February. p. 9.

Lucas, R., and L. Miller. 1981. The Evolution of Abortion Law in North America. *In* Abortion and Sterilization: Medical and Social Aspects. J.E. Hodgson, ed. New York: Grune & Stratton.

Luker, K. 1984a. The War Between the Women. Family Planning Perspectives 16:105–110.

———. 1984b. Abortion and the Politics of Motherhood. Berkeley: University of California Press.

Mayer, C. 1988. 800 rally against abortion. The Philadelphia Inquirer, 6 July.

Means, C. 1968. The Law of New York Concerning Abortion and the Status of the Foetus, 1664-1968: A Case of Cessation of Constitutionality. New York Law Forum 14: 411–515.

———. 1971. The Phoenix of Abortional Freedom: Is a Penumbral or Ninth Amendment Right about to Arise from the Nineteenth Century Legislative Ashes of a Fourteenth Century Common Law Liberty? New York Law Forum 17: 335–410.

Medawar, P.B. 1960. The Future of Man. New York: Basic Books.

Merton, A. 1981. Enemies of Choice. Boston: Beacon Press.

Mohr, James C. 1978. Abortion in America: The Origins and Evolution of National Policy. New York: Oxford University Press.

Nag, M. 1976. Factors Affecting Human Fertility in Nonindustrial Societies. New Haven: HRAF.

National Abortion Federation. 1988. Internal report.

New York Times. 1988. Text of Reagan's Address to nation on the State of the Union. 26 January, p. 10.

Obmascik, M. 1986. Right to Life group potent political force. The Denver Post, 15 June. p. 1.

Pear, R. 1988. Reagan bars mention of abortion at clinics receiving U.S. money. New York Times, 30 January. p. 1.

Peel, J., and M. Potts. 1969. Textbook of Contraceptive Practice. Cambridge: Cambridge University Press.

Petchesky, R.P. 1984. Abortion and Woman's Choice: The State, Sexuality, and Reproductive Freedom. Boston: Northeastern University Press.

Putnam, C. 1985a. Pro-Life: "Most feared" activist at CU. Colorado Daily, 18 October. p. 16.

———. 1985b. "Pro-Life" Picket: Anti-abortion activists "win" at Boulder clinic. Colorado Daily, 23 October.

Reagan R. 1984. Abortion and the Conscience of the Nation. Nashville: Thomas Nelson Publishers.

Reed, Robert. 1963. Arkansas Gazette, August 13.

Roberts, J. 1985. Abortion foe's picketing effort for naught; clinic shut for day. Denver Post, 23 October.

Robey, R. 1988. Shots fired at Boulder abortion clinic. The Denver Post, 6 February.

Rochat, R.R., et al. 1988. Maternal Mortality in the United States: Report from the Maternal Mortality Collaborative. Obstetrics and Gynecolology 72:91–97.

Rocky Mountain News. 1987. 21 November.

Roe v. Wade, 410 U.S. 113, 149 (1973).

Roemer, R. 1973. Legalization of Abortion in the United States. In The Abortion Experience. H.J. Osofsky and J.D. Osofsky, eds. Hagerstown: Harper and Row.

Romm, M. 1967. In Abortion in America. H. Rosen, ed. Boston: Beacon Press.

Scheidler, J.M. 1985. Closed: 99 Ways to Stop Abortion. Westchester: Il., Crossway Books.

Schmidt, W.E. 1986. Republicans court Iowa abortion foes. New York Times, 13 September.

Smothers R. 1988. Abortion protest grows in Atlanta. New York Times, 13 August. p. 1.

Tietze, C. 1984. The Public Health Effects of Legal Abortion in the United States. Family Planning Perspectives 16:26–28.

Tuchman, Barbara. 1978. A Distant Mirror. New York: Knopf.

UPI. 1981. Abortion foes meet with Reagan after march in capital. New York Times, 23 January. p. A 14.

Washington Times. Terrorist bombings decline; Abortion attacks excluded. 5 December, p. A4.

9

The Politics of Adolescent Pregnancy: Turf and Teens in Louisiana

Martha C. Ward

Many people in America believe that a serious "problem of teenage pregnancy" exists. A smaller number of them work actively to "solve the problem of teenage pregnancy." I do not intend to present the familiar picture of adolescent childbearing as a social problem in American society, to argue its "epidemic" status, or to recommend strategies for amelioration or prevention. My goal is to describe and analyze the cultural definitions and responses to the "problem," acting as an anthropologist in the role of participant-observer. I want to delineate the differences between ideal and real, to decipher the "messages" passed, and to explicate the cognitive structures of groups of care-givers or gate-keepers who have staked out their territories in the "problem."

Methods and Background

In formal interviews during the last three years I asked professionals who defined themselves as working in this field a series of major questions: What is the "problem"? Who or what defines it? Who or what causes it? What are their personal or agency goals in changing the "problem" (prevention, social change, public policy, personal empowerment)?[1]

The professionals interviewed represent approximately twenty public, private, religious, national and local agencies which have published agendas for dealing with the problems of adolescent pregnancy.[2]

The culture area under study is Louisiana with its major urban area, New Orleans. Without belaboring the litany of depressing statistics, suffice it to say that Louisiana is at the top of most lists of social pathologies and bottom of the list for health and human services. Louisiana is third in the nation in the number of live births to teenagers (adolescents are defined as 19 and under). Twenty-four percent of the over 13,000 births were second and third pregnancies. The extent of sexual activity is reflected by the statistic that 30 percent of the reported cases of syphilis and gonorrhea were among adolescents.[3]

The statistics on teen pregnancy parallels what we already know about rural areas or poor port cities in the rest of America (Hayes 1987). Rates of adolescent pregnancy combined with infant mortality, school-leaving, unemployment, or associated factors are among the highest, if not the highest, in the nation. In Orleans Parish one out of eight females age 15 to 19 is currently pregnant. For 1985, the infant mortality rate was 50 percent higher than the national rate (16.4 per 1000 live births in Orleans Parish versus 10.6 nationwide). One out of every four low birthweight babies is born to a young mother. Ninety percent of pregnant teens drop out of school and the school board believes that eighty percent of them will never return.

One major set of facts is crucial. New Orleans is a black majority city and all public or educational programming starts with that fact.

The Models

Policy-makers, educators, care-providers, and other gatekeepers have explanations (and reinforcing statistics) for what they perceive as "the problem," "the cause," and "the cure." It is possible to group these cognitive or explanatory models into major categories. Group members spend significant amounts of time and resources on the socialization of each other into the assumptions of their models. Although they use fragments of other models on occasion, their gut reactions and deeply held values are apparent when they are pushed (as in heated public debates or key political stands). In each of these models, identifiable political corollaries or outcomes spring from the postulates of the model. Proponents of each model identify themselves with key phrases or "buzzwords." All groups are linked to national organizations; therefore, no "local" or uniquely Louisianan cause or cure is proposed. The groups are also linked to national identities like race, gender, class, religion, or ethnicity, although they rarely spell out this consciousness.

The following categories or models predominate when professionals discuss the issues of teen pregnancy or when they develop programs.

The Nature of Teenagers

The first model or working category for adolescent childbearing is the adolescent development model. This consists of a series of agreements emerging from contemporary psychology and education. The answer to the questions of what causes the phenomenon or what intervention programs should be made starts with such a typical statement as "you have to understand what teenagers are like." They are said to be influenced by hormones, early menarche, peer pressure, and the media while exhibiting personality characteristics summarized by concepts such as rebelliousness, narcissism, passivity, poor self-esteem, and unrealistic fantasies. Teenagers are a psychologically, physiologically, and socially unique age grade according to these theories. Variations of these theories will be found in our best scientific literature and in the folklore or lay analysis throughout this country. Just ask the parent of any teenager for the conventional wisdom.

The key words for translating these theories into action are motivation and self-esteem. "We need to educate these young people to a healthy sexual attitude, a sense of their own uniqueness, beauty and worth, and an understanding of their bodies." (Interview at the Family Life Apostolate). This will be accomplished through "family life education"— the buzzword for a rationalist philosophical stance in which people (read adolescents) will act in enlightened self-interest once they have been properly taught, educated, or socialized in the truth. Once they understand the consequences of their actions, they will maximize their potential like the "rational man" who dominated economic theory for so long. The socialization model assumes that better and better educational techniques will produce the desired result, that is, an approximation to the national adult reproductive model or the middle-class, heterosexual familial model.

In the adolescent development model, teenagers can be and must be reached by education. Health services, particularly contraceptive services and availability of birth control technology, are taken as a given. In fact, this model assumes that teenagers know more about sex, pregnancy, intercourse and birth control than they know about their own feelings and motivations. They are either unaware of their own motivations, have the wrong motivations, or need to be motivated. The conventional wisdom is that they do not practice what they hear preached.

The programmatic trick is to insure even more sex education at earlier ages. The liberal margin of this approach will be found in the so-called "life planning curriculas" (such as the Center for Population Options or the national family planning associations endorse). In these curriculas the emphasis is on the meaning of a teen's whole life—jobs, careers, educational achievement, self-esteem, and personal relationships. Teachers put the anatomy and physiology of reproduction (the "plumbing") or birth control in its place—in a larger life context.

The ultimate goal of these programs is to train cadres of professionals who work with adolescents. In this view, it is too difficult to mount programs for a cohort of adolescents who change rapidly in a six to ten year passage through the dangerous years. Evaluation research on the long range effectiveness of these programs is very expensive, rarely conducted, and inconclusive (Hayes 1987).

The Nature of Society

The second model which I have isolated in the field of adolescent pregnancy debates is what we could call "the social-structural model." This model is based not on assumption of individuals making decisions and planning their lives, but of key groups in American society acted on by social and historical forces which are themselves pathological. The underlying political assumptions are that any solutions will have to be found in some radical restructuring of the economic-work-reward system for American society. This model is about class and color.

You will see this model when a meeting of professionals concerned about the issue begins with statements such as:

- We have to put racism on the table. Racism is the real problem.
- I am committing money and energy to this problem, because the crime situation is getting out of hand in New Orleans.
- If the business community wants to help, then they can provide jobs for those boys.

The most elaborated examples of this model come from males who typically approach the "problem of teen pregnancy" from the point of view of economic development, the cycle of poverty, illiteracy, and welfare costs. The "solutions" will include such programs as preventing school dropouts, providing job training, restructuring welfare, and increasing the government's responsibility to all its citizens. Within the model, there is a very sharp difference between the black view and the white view.

The black socio-structural model, when in use, centers on economic opportunities (jobs, education, and social mobility). Implicit is the assumption that white men are faulting black men for not taking care of women and children. This is a defense against the statistics which show large numbers of black female-headed household and infants born out of wedlock. The answer for black males is more economic opportunities for black males; the provider status depends upon employment. Institutionalized racism is the ultimate cause of the chain which begins in lack of jobs and ends in high black infant mortality figures. The statistics for whites in adolescent pregnancy and growing rates of poor single parent families are dismissed.

In this black model, the fighting word is population. In the words of the Director of the New Orleans Welfare Department and president of the National Association of Black Social Workers:

> I think reproduction patterns are based on self-interest, although not in any conscious sense. And when you look at the gains the black community has made, it hasn't been based so much on opportunity as on the profoundness of numbers. In the political arena, you count votes. My contention is that you can have both large numbers and a high quality of life, but it's predicated on reforms in the economic system and in the public policy arena. The best self-interest of the black community is for it to have its numbers. I could not support a position that we should decrease our numbers. This is what Darwin was talking about. Concern about teenage pregnancy is couched in terms of concern for the black community. But why is the white community all of a sudden concerned about the quality of life in the black community? (*Times-Picayune,* October 7, 1987: A-9.)

The phrase "let's put the real agenda on the table" marks much of the public discourse about teenage pregnancy for black politics. Black politicians and professionals regularly express skepticism about the attention generated by the issue of teenage pregnancy and wonder whether the mandate is to minister to the needy or to cut off the population spigot.

Many leading black professionals state their views that population policy, certain economic policies, and programs for adolescent pregnancy are, in fact, a "hidden white agenda." In private interviews, the fears of genocide are openly discussed. The word itself rarely appears in the press except in coded form such as the statement quoted above. At the regular conferences and task force meetings held on the subject, white leaders will go to elaborate lengths to dissuade their black colleagues that genocide is not the population policy of either the U.S. government or the state of Louisiana.

Genocide appears to be an important code word not for blacks' perceptions of a racial holocaust or concentration camps as a racist white policy, but for the lack of economic opportunities and institutionalized racism particularly for urban black males. This is why the Urban League, which falls squarely in this model, sponsors a number of national programs for what they call "male responsibility" or "male motivation." This may also account for their lack of enthusiasm about sex education in schools as a solution for the problems (however they are defined).

The key concepts are "local option," or community standards, and the involvement of organized religion.

> Local communities and religious organizations should develop systems for development, coordination, and implementation of existing and needed services aimed at the reduction of early adolescent pregnancy and early sexual intercourse including, but not limited to, the school environment (Delta Assembly recommendations p. 11).

The political sequelae of this social structure approach is complicated because it must hope for or presuppose an antidote to racism and poverty. There is also a double-bind inherent in these approaches. Blacks do not wish to be cast as either the cause (as when the statistics show black-white differences) or as the victims. Hence the assertions that teenage pregnancy is not a problem, only a symptom of much larger problems. On the other hand, any public programs specifically addressed to the issue of teenage pregnancy, certainly in Louisiana, must be skewed to the black agenda.

The white social-structural model is built on the ideal of "the quality of urban life." At the conservative end of the spectrum, the concrete concerns are crime, the cycle of poverty, or the availability of trained and willing workers for industries and businesses such as the tourism. The liberal end of the spectrum will emphasize the rates of infant mortality (twice as high for blacks as for whites), good prenatal care, and the now voluminous documentation about the relationships of age at first pregnancy, family size, educational achievement, career development, and social mobility. These statistics are regularly cited as the reason for "doing something about teenage pregnancy," which is seen as the structural cause of many problems of urban life.

Proponents of this position will often advocate mandatory sex education programs, liberal abortion policies, or welfare reform. They believe that the state and local governments have a serious economic stake—a developmental responsibility—for solving the "problem." Coalitions of groups along this continuum may be found lobbying the legislature and the City Council as issues arise.

Both black and white proponents of this socio-structural model see various social pathologies as causative. In their menu of the evils leading to unwed mothers and unfathered babies, they may see any or all of the following: divorce, working mothers, day care, poor teachers, poor schools, the rise of feminism, or parental permissiveness.

The Nature of Being Female

Another important set of models focus on what women are like. While these viewpoints are not necessarily feminist, they are most visible in their black and white forms. The "female-focused" model may share some of the same assumptions with either of the other models, but it is primarily characterized by an emphasis on woman as actors. Proponents of these models tend to be defensive about interpreting the statistics on female-headed households and unwed motherhood as social pathology.

The literature in social science on kin-centered domestic networks and female-headed households is particularly instructive for teenage pregnancy (Stack 1975; Ladner 1971). As we have learned, economic conditions create adaptations in which public assistance (welfare, AFDC, food stamps) go to women with children. Since this money provides only bare necessities of food and rent, the domestic networks exchange services and practice reciprocity, economic interdependence and mutual obligations. Residence patterns are elastic and the motto is "blood is thicker than water."

The surest form of admission to and continued support from these groups is a baby. Pregnancy and childbirth may also be seen as an initiation or rite of passage into adulthood for adolescent females. Child-care is a kin obligation, rather than an obligation limited to a nuclear male-headed household or single individual. Following this logic, it is easy to see some very powerful motives for pregnancy. Having a baby, even at a very young age, is the link to support networks, and one of the few routes to validation and adult status. If a young girl sees no routes out of poverty, then she must maximize her chances within the system. Welfare money or a low paying job will not support herself and a baby, but will bind the domestic network to her and insure her status.

Simultaneously, no one sees advantages in customs of marriage when men have even less access to economic resources. Supporting a husband or lover is not adequate and may separate a woman from more advantageous support networks. There is a strong statistical possibility that his maternal relatives will be drawn into the kin networks of their brother, son, or grandson. A girl's mother, grandmother or other female relatives can be counted on to provide fosterage—"child-keeping" or "bringing up" in the vernacular (Stack 1975).

As Lancaster and Hamburg observe, there is "an important subgroup of urban, poor, black adolescents who are choosing early childbearing as an alternative life course which promotes their social and cultural survival and enhances personal development" (1986:7). If, as for many blacks in Louisiana and elsewhere, adolescence and early adulthood is a part of the life cycle characterized by high unemployment and lack of job opportunities, they will still benefit from an institutionalization of the domestic, familial, and informal networks of support. In these cases, the outcomes of early pregnancy are not always dismal, but success depends almost entirely on the presence of support systems.

This view of the causes and consequences of teen pregnancy is vociferously supported by black women I interviewed in Louisiana. They may phrase their analysis as "we take care of our own," "it's the work of the Lord," or "most of my friends and relatives have babies." They speak of the value of babies and the joys of having children. This analysis also partially explains (as they point out) the low incidence of either abortion or adoption among black teens. A type of program they emphasize is education, training and seminars for adult women—the relatives of adolescents—to prepare them and give them the necessary background to do sex education in their own homes. They want to emphasize the role of churches as primary educators because they see community and family values as the causative and curative factor. They would be happy if teenagers chose to delay pregnancy, but are not willing to judge the mother too harshly.

Although this model of teen pregnancy has probably the most anthropological coherence, it is poorly represented in new legislation in Louisiana or in task force reports whose formal goals are centered on prevention or economic development. The chief political efforts by groups which follow this model will be concentrated in extending the social support systems for women and children even more broadly. This will include advocacy for child care, day care, broader and more accessible medical and maternal-child health services, and welfare reform on female-focused lines. The National Council for Negro Women, Child-Watch, and several strong black sororities, among others, are the types of organizations which fall into this category.

The second major group in the "female-focused" category is best represented by white women who are veterans of the woman's movement (politically and personally). They center their educational, advocacy, and financial efforts on female sexuality as the issue. They speak not of "sex education" but emphatically of "sexuality education." As the intellectual descendants of Margaret Sanger, they find value in quality love-making, committed relationships, and birth control as an expression of selfhood and decision-making. They perceive adolescent females as making a series of decisions about their sexuality. Sex should be fun and linked to pregnancy and marriage only by conscious decisions. To make these choices and to maximize "sexuality," girls need education programs which offer the carrot of independence, mobility, and sensuality.

Politically, this stance translates into programs which enhance parent-child communication skills, a feminist or at least female-centered, personalized health care. The word "choice" is particularly important to these women. Although for some this word is synonymous with abortion availability, it also exemplifies choosing sexuality and birth control. This translates to a deep concern for but uneasy relationship with adolescent pregnancy. Girls are seen as decision-makers, as actors in their own destiny. Adults are seen as facilitators—clearing the way through complex sets of services, legislation, and education. In this theory, knowledge is empowering, education is freeing.

Proponents of this approach will find themselves advocating mandatory sexuality education, the various "life planning" curricula, full confidentiality and availability for all women (including adolescents) to contraceptive care, sexually transmitted disease diagnosis and treatment, and abortion (including government funded abortions for poor women). They will be against the so-called "squeal rule," or other legislatively imposed sanctions against sexual activity or its consequences for women. Groups which fall into this category (for at least part of their programs) include the Planned Parenthood Federation of America, American Civil Liberties Union, National Organization for Women and their coalitions for reproductive freedoms.

At the margins they will work for any other reforms which affect women (rape, incest, battered wives, day-care, welfare reform, gay rights, and medical confidentiality.) Their philosophical assumption is that adolescent females are, by definition, adult women in their sexual and reproductive functions. Although uncomfortable with the notions of abstinence and chastity, they will advocate any practice and mechanisms which delay intercourse and pregnancy.

The Nature of Being Religious

The most powerful force to be reckoned with in programs for pregnant teenagers are the organized religious structures and the belief systems of many people that religious groups hold programs hostage to their own agendas. Louisiana has the second largest diocese in America and New Orleans is a Catholic city with membership and influence which cut widely across class and color lines. In conducting research on family planning and teen pregnancy, I regularly encounter the assumption that the Church's position is monolithic and conservative. This may be true elsewhere and is certainly true for what we can call "the Magisterium" (the male international policy makers—symbolized by the Pope).

Extensive interviewing and analysis, however, show another side of Catholic policy for those professionals directly involved in delivery of services and education. Historically in Louisiana, the Catholic church restrained their opposition to the United States' largest family planning program (Ward 1986) and issued public statements that "we do not support but we will not oppose." That stated policy, begun in the early 1960s, remains solidly in effect. However, Catholic laypersons and non-Catholics alike hold a set of folk beliefs about Catholicism. Their "conventional wisdom" is that the political and theological power of the Church remains arrayed solidly against even the whisper of birth control, prevention programs, or even a frank discussion of sexual techniques.

The bureaucratic truth is that, through the 1970s and 1980s, Catholic agencies have to confront the social consequences of adolescent child-bearing more directly than any other set of bureaucracies in the state. Their outreach efforts center on an enormous parochial school system, three Catholic colleges (one black), and a social services system larger than the city or parish agencies. Caregivers and educators perceive themselves as picking up the pieces with a wide variety of programs in food, shelter, medical care, counseling, family disintegration, and infant morbidity.

The Catholic charity bureaucracy used to manage residential programs for pregnant teens with corollary programs for adoption. This was an uphill battle as only seven percent of teenagers choose to adopt out their babies, so these residential programs have been closed. Since most of the pregnant teens choose to keep their babies and remain unmarried, elaborate efforts in child-rearing training and social supports for single parenting are necessary and expensive. The majority of programs in Louisiana for mothers and infants are mounted by, staffed by, or supported by Catholics.

Torn between an ethic of caregiving for seriously expanding needs and practical solutions in prevention officially prohibited, many Catholic professionals have opted for positions which narrowly skirt the borders of ecclesiastical legality. For example, the parochial schools regularly invite such organizations as Planned Parenthood to give seminars in schools and churches. The scope of these is limited only by the resources of the Planned Parenthood personnel. Elaborate curricula in "family life education" are more widely used in parochial schools than in public schools (such curriculum simply omit mention of contraceptives but place heavy emphasis on self-esteem, decision-making, and family formation). I have heard lectures which begin with the statement, "Here are the major forms of medically approved birth control—which you are not supposed to use, and the places you can get help—which you are not supposed to go to." Associated Catholic Charities and some prominent Catholic institutions have also quietly severed their connections to Right-to-Life (an antiabortion group).

At conferences or task force meetings on the problems of teenage pregnancy, Catholic participation is careful but complete. Catholic officials may object to the word "choice" (the association with the word abortion is too strong). They usually request that family planning be presented as voluntary and private so they do not have to endorse officially. Prenatal and postnatal care for all women is a stronger value than preventive care. In this concern they find allies in the blacks who fear population control through involuntary control of pregnancy.

Comprehensive, culturally relevant family planning and postnatal services should be made available to all who desire them. The need for everyone to be aware of such services and their importance in any pregnancy decision should be emphasized. The services and programs provided should always provide for local option (Delta Assembly 1987:11).

The head of the Associated Catholic Charities (a nun), the head of the Archdioceses Schools (a Catholic layperson), and a prominent monsignor, outlined their evolving approach in "family life education." It is proper to teach about and recognize all forms of what they call "sexual activity." Under this rubric is petting, necking, masturbation, fantasy, mutual play, or whatever, but not vaginal intercourse. Intercourse is strictly for marriage and making babies. This makes possible the acknowledgement of sex outside of marriage and the sexual nature of humans while still upholding the ban on what they call "artificial birth control." They also teach the Billings method or the rhythm method. This message of human sexuality bears little relationship to what the layperson or general public thinks that Catholics are doing. In fact, these philosophies are carefully stated by key policy makers who claim to spend more time educating their own laypeople than they do training teenagers.

The opposite end of the religious spectrum are the "fundamentalists." This includes conservative Protestants, spiritual churches, some legislators from northern Louisiana, tiny religious groups who picket the abortion clinics, and others who bring no overarching organization to their generalized platform. They can be counted to oppose sex education in schools and to endorse "values" and "morality." They are seen as the power behind the restrictive sex education laws in Louisiana which prohibit classroom instruction below the seventh grade and limit severely the character of instruction for middle and high schools. Groups with more liberal agendas fear this undifferentiated power. Even one vocal individual with powerful political contacts can sabotage or destroy programs.

The Nature of Being Sexual

When we factor out the questions in the teenage pregnancy debate about who sets policy, who pays for services, what kind of services and who should receive the attention, the underlying issue becomes what is sex, who should get it, and who should pay the price for it. The real dilemma for policy makers is the nature of sex itself.

For example, it is ironic that the liberal margins of Catholic education about sexuality also parallels the recommendations of sex therapists both locally and nationally, the safer sex guidelines promoted by the various AIDS groups, the national family planning establishment, and the female-focused groups discussed above. This makes sex or sexual activity or sexuality an age-appropriate or age-graded process. It takes the question of the validity, the fallibility, or the availability of contraception out of the discussion.

The nature of human sexuality and whether we can or should control it is the key question for those who use the developmental explanatory model. What are teenagers really doing? What models for sexual behavior do they have? Are the models appropriate for different class or ethnic groups? Assuming that a philosophy for sexual activity is suitable for females, is it suitable for males? Is education a sufficient tool for diffusing an energy of the type that fuels adolescent pregnancy? None of the professionals ever said that the fundamental cause of pregnancy was sperm; no one mentions that the delivery system for sperm is called boys.

Recently, AIDS has added a new dimension to this discussion for all of the groups mentioned above. Many public discussions escape talking about sex as connected to adolescent pregnancy; but there is no escaping the linkage of HIV infection to sex and drugs. There are new coalitions focusing on sexual activity and the so-called "safe sex" guidelines as applied to teenage groups at risk. When I first started interviewing, AIDS was not a part of professional consciousness or public programming. It is now, although the situation parallels the scene for adolescent pregnancy. The messages are tentative and painful; the programs are fragmented; and public attention is uncoordinated. In Louisiana, as nationally, there are no statewide programs.

The various safer-sex guidelines will probably become the new taboo system (rivaling anything anthropologists ever studied before). But communicating information about AIDS (and sexually transmitted diseases) to teenagers means that we must assume a prior knowledge of sexual anatomy, physiology, techniques, positions and alternative life-styles. These latter domains of information are part of very few "sex education" programs in America and certainly not in Louisiana. In fact, evidence indicates that such information is not always possessed by adults who decide policy or by parents (Hayes 1987).

The Nature of Being "Savages"

The other golden thread which runs through this research is the treatment of adolescents as "the new savages." Adults are worried about or believe in the potentially pathological world view of this specific subculture. Responsible people must provide the services, socialization, and motivation for "the others" to change and embrace a life style which is believed to make them happier or, at least, to cease causing problems for us. In the past we heard the voices of colonial administrators, religious practitioners, policy makers and developers who wished to bring enlightenment to the Third World. Now the government, adults, parents and teachers are supposed to carry out the task of converting these new savages.

Not a single person I have interviewed espoused what anthropologists regard as one of the cornerstones of our methodology—the emic approach. No one suggested talking to the "native speakers" to find out what was really going on. All the professionals, educators, or agents of social change have very precise theories of why and how adolescents act, but all of it is based on outsider experiences and their own memories of being a teen. There are, of course, surveys on attitudes and perceptions. But there are no grammars, no analyses of world views. This is an interesting omission in groups who take on the goal of changing another group.

Few of the agencies contacted has as part of its agenda the victimization of teenagers. No one suggested that coercion, through rape or incest, might be a systematic factor in eleven year-old children getting pregnant. No agencies had organized support for fathers—particularly when unmarried to their babies' mothers. The ambiguity about adolescents' legal status (are they adults or minors?) warps the debates about what to do about the problems they cause. None of the curricula, programs, video, or presentations discussed homosexuality as a choice—such is the force of the assumptions of "family life education."

Imagine that you are a teenager. Accept as given the media messages and other major socializing influences over which public programming has no influence. In Louisiana sex education is allowed in only seven out of sixty-four parishes and is prohibited completely below the seventh grade. There are no comprehensive training or certification programs for teachers. Public school personnel like counselors and nurses are prohibited from making referrals for students seeking information. There is a state family planning program which can handle only welfare and other federally supported programs such as Medicaid. The wait for an appointment is many months. Education and counseling for individuals is perfunctory at best. Planned Parenthood has only one small, three-year old clinic. It is difficult to argue that contraceptives are widely available. Given the poverty of the state, private doctors are out of the question (and most are unwilling to serve poor adolescents).

Sometimes I am reminded of the debates in anthropology earlier in this century about whether "natives" really know where babies came from. In Malinowski's great classic, *The Sexual Life of Savages* (1929), he argues the case for the Trobriand Islanders' misconceptions about the relationship between intercourse and the birth of babies. He is convinced that the islanders willfully refuse the truth that sperm and egg equally cause pregnancy, preferring to believe in the reality of the Baloma spirits in conception. It is possible to analyze the current debates by casting American adolescents as the "new savages." Do they actually understand the relationship of sperm and egg or are they acting on a wider social agenda of their own in which the petty action of biology is inconsequential? Most of the debate, regardless of which camp we favor, centers on convincing these others to accept our world view.

Adolescents are the "new savages" in another respect. They are transitional, economically marginal, liminal, unorganized, acephalous, and politically powerless. They have no national association for their social interests or the promotion of the age grade (by sharp contrast with senior citizens, the American Association for Retired People, Gray Panthers, and the vast social security-Medicare apparatus). They are savages in that their sexuality is believed to be rampant and uncontrolled, a threat to the body politic. Underlying the welfare reform controversies is a belief that uncontrolled females and their fertility can force extraordinary amounts of social resources in their direction with individual passivity. Urban males—thought of as jobless, producing babies for trophies, and mired in gangs, drugs, and crime—are the modern Indians who had to be dealt with before the frontier was civilized.

Teenagers are seen as creating many of the problems of poverty, schools, and being the chief barrier to the promise of urbanization and the quality of life. The phenomenon of female-headed households which frequently start as unwed pregnancies are widely heralded as a form of social pathology and a sign of the breakdown of family life in America.

Being Political

The turf battles that result from the lack of goals or methods are best seen in a recent controversy over school-based clinics. The parish health department which has not even been able to provide minimal prenatal care has received a mandate to develop a model school clinic with a hope (though not directly stated) of reducing teen pregnancies. The legendary black ghetto called Desire (the largest housing project in America) was selected as a site and a national grant submitted. The Desire project has all the characteristics of social pathology statistically associated with teen pregnancy, infant mortality, morbidity, and has been a frequent target of ameliorative programs.

The first controversy, still unresolved, was the provision of birth control (pills and condoms). Several powerful black legislators are opposed to the idea of school based clinics, the provision of contraceptives to women, or the mention of certain tabooed topics. Other black organizations have entered the fray to contend that they have the most experience (however they define that) in dealing with adolescents and should be the preferred vendor. Some of these organizations argue that health care is not the issue at all. Liberal organizations like Planned Parenthood are privately distressed because they claim that the delivery of health care services to adolescents is a complicated issue in which parish-city agencies have no experience or background. The grant was funded but the school board has refused to cooperate and the public arguments remain unsolved.

The ultimate controversies are over political control, access to whatever money is available, which groups get the credit from their constituencies, which groups receive the blame, and, when the dust settles on occasion, what is the problem anyway. The agencies with whom I interviewed continue to produce pamphlets, programs, task forces, public statements, videos, and lectures. Only a few provide direct services (health care, physical examinations, referrals, contraceptives, childcare, job training, compensatory education, housing, or emergency aid). Most offer advice and counseling to people who have not asked or advocacy on behalf of groups they have never spoken to.

These groups constantly realign themselves in coalitions, task forces, conferences, or transition teams. They write position papers, solicit grant money, and do "networking" (sometimes a buzzword for intelligence finding—CIA style). What are the "other sides" up to? How can we protect our investment and our turf? Ostensibly these networks and taskforces are to share information, develop coalitions, and promote advocacy. But it is difficult for those who want to discuss female sexuality and choice to communicate with those who believe that the United States has a genocidal policy for blacks.

When I asked professionals in the agencies, "what is the bottom line?," they replied, "We have to communicate with teenagers." Education is the answer. But the messages they want to send are baffling: Delay intercourse as long as possible. But when you do it, do it with protection.

Don't have sex until you are married to someone who hasn't had sex either. You can do anything but intercourse. That's for marriage and babies. Sex is beautiful-fun-fulfilling. Know your partner. Use condoms. Communicate. Just say no.

The chief value expressed in the cultures of the professionals was "we have to help them, show them the way, educate them, and bring them into our value system." But the program goals of the major agencies (public and private) are fragmented. No cohort of adolescents are systematically reached by any of the program under study. None of the programs at the local, state or national level has a "lever" for institutional change. The messages are confusing, conflicting, or relevant only under highly structured circumstances. There are no external incentives for teenagers to comply with or to participate in what might be perceived as the value system of a foreign culture (middle class adulthood). A pregnant adolescent is perceived as a threat to herself, her future, her baby, her family and, ultimately, to the good of society.

Whatever the apparent divisiveness of the problem of teenage pregnancy, the professionals who care about the solutions are united by an uncommon pain. The topic of teenage pregnancy forces civic and personal anxieties as few topics can. The touched nerves in a serious interview will inevitably include: the worries of parenting, drugs, educational failures and policies, crime, death, disease, poverty, class, abortion, adoption, race, sex and the connections between all of these. This public and private pain has forced yet another coalition out of the Mayor's office in 1988. After extensive debate a new "Let's Talk" campaign, modeled after successes in other cities, had been inaugurated with a consortium of 180 civic and community agencies including the Catholic Archdiocese, Planned Parenthood, black neighborhood associations, black professional organizations, and every parish, state, and national group with a stated concern for adolescent pregnancy.

The largest arena of agreement is that sexual activity for teenagers should be postponed ("encourage them to delay sexual activity"). The second arena of agreement is that information about contraceptives should be provided to adolescents. There have been many other programs for teenage pregnancy prevention. The initial victory for the "Let's Talk" campaign is that the organizations whose philosophies are described above have stated their willingness to listen to each other.

Notes

1. I have access to publications, minutes of meetings, grant applications, clients, and other resources for understanding the problem. In March of 1987, the University of New Orleans School of Urban and Regional Studies and the

American Assembly of Columbia University invited seventy professionals primarily from Louisiana and Mississippi to the Delta Regional Assembly in Biloxi, Mississippi, for a conference. Although a broad range of topics on the agenda included the economic issues of population growth, community support systems, and parenting, the emotional focus of the conference was adolescent pregnancy. Attending the conference as a participant and observer was a culmination and confirmation of previous research.

2. The professional groups interviewed include: Associated Catholic Charities (Access Pregnancy and Referral Center, St. Vincent's Maternity Medical Clinic); Archdiocesan Office of the Social Apostolate; Charity Hospital (New Horizons Unit; Women's Outpatient Clinic); United Teachers of New Orleans (American Federation of Teachers); Urban League (Adolescent Prevention Program; Parent Child Center); Planned Parenthood of Louisiana (Planned Parenthood Federation of America); Human Resources, Policy and Planning (Office of the Mayor, City Hall); National Council of Negro Women of Greater New Orleans, Inc.; League of Women Voters; National Organization for Women (Reproductive Rights Task Force); YWCA (Pregnancy Prevention for Teens); Vincent Memorial Legacy (Episcopal Diocese Offices); Louisiana State Family Planning Program; Association of School Nurses (New Orleans, Louisiana); Sex and Marital Health Clinic (Louisiana State University Medical Center); Child Watch; American Civil Liberties Union; Orleans Parish School Board; Alliance for Human Services; Greater New Orleans Foundation; United Way; Orleans Parish Medical Society; Black Women Physicians' Organization; Kingsley House; Covenant House.

3. The statistics quoted here are taken from the Alan Guttmacher Institute, Louisiana Office of Vital Statistics, Charity Hospital, the Office of Employment of the Louisiana Department of Labor, and the Orleans Parish School Board. I am grateful for the assistance of the personnel of these agencies as well as those professionals in the above agencies who graciously talked to me.

References Cited

Center for Population Options. 1985. Life Planning Education: A Youth Development Program. Washington, D.C.

Delta Assembly. 1987. The Population Issue. Final Statement. University of New Orleans: School of Urban and Regional Studies.

Hayes, Cherytl D. (ed.). 1987. National Research Council. Risking the Future: Adolescent Sexuality, Pregnancy, and Childbearing. Washington, D.C.: National Academy Press.

Ladner, Joyce A. 1971. Tomorrow's Tomorrow: The Black Woman. Garden City, New York: Doubleday.

Lancaster, J.B., and B. Hamburg (eds.). 1986. School-Age Pregnancy and Parenthood: Biosocial Perspectives. New York: Aldine.

Malinowski, Bronislaw. 1929. The Sexual Life of Savages. New York: Harcourt, Brace and World, Inc.

Mullener, Elizabeth. 1987. Poverty's Children: Solutions to Teenage Pregnancy. New Orleans Times-Picayune October 4,5,6,7. Page 1.

New Orleans Public Schools. 1984. Task Force on Adolescent Pregnancy. Co-Sponsored by the Mott Foundation. Presented to the City of New Orleans.

Stack, Carol. B. 1975. All Our Kin: Strategies for Survival in a Black Community. New York: Harper.

State of Louisiana. 1985. Report of the Governor's Commission on Children and Youth. April. Troubled Systems: A Blueprint for Change.

Ward, Martha C. 1986. Poor Women, Powerful Men: America's Great Experiment in Family Planning. Boulder, Colo.: Westview Press.

10

The Politics of Family Planning: Sterilization and Human Rights in Bangladesh

Barbara Pillsbury

In 1985 the population and family planning program in Bangladesh catapulted into controversy at the highest policy-making levels in Washington, D.C., and West European capitals. For many years, family planning programs in Bangladesh and other developing countries were strongly supported by a decided constituency of U.S. government policy-makers. From other Washington, D.C., policy-makers, the subject had evinced only dreary ho-hums; many of the latter were not much interested in either Bangladesh or family planning and often dismissed the country as a hopeless basketcase anyway. In 1985, however, many Congressmen and others became understandably concerned about charges that the major U.S.-funded foreign aid donors to the Bangladesh family planning program—the United States Agency for International Development (A.I.D.), the World Bank, and the United Nations Fund for Population Assistance (UNFPA)—supported policies that were coercive, even illegal, and that fundamental human rights were being violated by the Bangladesh program.

Women in Bangladesh were undergoing forced sterilizations. At least, so said the critics.

Ironically, feminist critics on the political left provided fuel for family planning opponents on the political right, most of whom are identified with the "New Right" movement in American politics (Reichley 1984). These right-wing critics tried to make sterilization in Bangladesh the next *cause célèbre*, after abortion in China, in their campaign to influence conservatives in the U.S. Congress to cut off more and ultimately all funding for international family planning assistance (with the exception of "natural family planning").[1]

This campaign was waged alongside of and was in fact closely linked to continuing attempts to cut off federal funding within the U.S. for abortion and even family planning in general (Congressional Record 1986). Indeed, the controversy over the Bangladesh family planning program can only be understood in the context of the conservative climate in the United States in the 1980s in which antiabortion groups are trying to restrict access to abortion and, ultimately, to overturn the historic 1973 Roe vs. Wade decision that legalized abortion in the U.S. more than a decade earlier.

What was the basis for these charges about Bangladesh? What is the reality? How did it happen that liberal feminists became aligned with right-to-lifers? What has been the outcome? This chapter answers these questions and hopes to provide a better understanding of the dangers that uninformed criticism poses for the well-being of women and families in the dire circumstances they often face in poor Third World countries. Conclusions presented here are based on intensive interviews, clinic and field visits (including unannounced visits, unaccompanied by officials, to clinics while sterilizations were being performed), and analysis of research findings and program documents in Bangladesh in 1980, 1981, and 1985; comparison with family planning programs in other countries where sterilization is available; and on interviews with A.I.D. officials and others in Washington, D.C. (See Pillsbury, Kangas, and Margolis 1981; Edmonds, Minkler, Pillsbury, and Bernhart 1985; and Pillsbury and Knowles 1986.) Interviews were conducted with a wide range of people, including many critics of the program. People interviewed included: Bangladeshi men and women who have been sterilized, men and women who use other methods of family planning, and men and women who use no family planning; clinic personnel and fieldworkers in the government-sponsored family planning program; managers, clinic personnel, and fieldworkers of family planning projects sponsored by non-governmental agencies (private and voluntary organizations); representatives of the United Nations and other bilateral donor agencies, including European donors and others that have been critical of the sterilization program; representatives of Bangladeshi women's groups that have expressed concern about women's needs and rights; social scientists and others who have been carrying out in-depth and survey research in rural Bangladesh; and officials in the Bangladesh government and at USAID/Dhaka, the Dhaka offices of the U.S. Agency for International Development.

Attack from the West

It was a phenomenon peculiar to the United States in the mid-1980s that the attacks on the Bangladesh family planning program—and the role of sterilization in it—came both from the American left and right. The charges against the Bangladesh program and the international aid donors that supported it ranged from ideological indictments ("waging an all-out war on the poor") to criticisms of the quality of clinical services. Critics alleged that human rights named in various U.N. declarations were being violated and that Bangladesh family planning personnel were engaging in activities that are illegal under the U.S. Foreign Assistance Act. Sterilization was at the heart of the attacks.

Two publications in particular had wide circulation and, through media coverage, considerable impact on the policy-making process. One was *The Deadly Neo-Colonialism*, issued and distributed in Washington, D.C., by Human Life International (O'Reilly 1985). The other was *Food, Saris, and Sterilization*, issued in London in mid-1985 by the Bangladesh International Action Group (Hartmann and Standing 1985), a group whose aims are "to campaign against violations of human rights, work to end the harmful activities of multinational companies in Bangladesh, and to expose the harmful effects of foreign aid." The authors of both publications made it clear that they wanted to close down the family planning program in Bangladesh or at least to force major structural changes. Their charges were repeated approvingly by the press in several donor countries and it appeared that they might well succeed.

The Deadly Neo-Colonialism was said to be based on a three-month investigation of the Bangladesh family planning program. In fact, the author, William O'Reilly, is neither a social scientist nor a medical, public health, or rural development specialist but a Washington, D.C., CPA who is untrained in the methods of investigation necessary to carry out such research. Furthermore, the author's three months in Bangladesh were as a financial analyst on assignment to the Asian Development Bank. Field trips and clinic visits made by the author were only ad hoc activities (Robinson 1985:9).

The Deadly Neo-Colonialism publication bristled with moral outrage. Its charges may be summarized as follows:

1. The family planning program in Bangladesh is coercive in nature; the use of financial reimbursements to sterilization clients amounts to financial coercion of the poor. The government is moving toward a "Chinese model" of population control using even more drastic means to reduce fertility.
2. The U.S. is financing such operations, directly through A.I.D. in Bangladesh and indirectly through the U.S. contributions to UNFPA and the World Bank.
3. The U.S. regulations against any financing of abortions or monetary incentives for family planning acceptance are "mostly symbolic"

and are ignored in practice by the donors and by the government of Bangladesh.

4. The program is largely controlled by the major donors who do not respect the religious and cultural values in Bangladesh. The program deliberately targets the poor, the hungry, and the Hindus.

Food, Saris, and Sterilization was written by authors who saw family planning and population control as part and parcel of the "World Bank-multinational-U.S.A.I.D. conspiracy" against the people of the Third World. This report was published in July 1985, just before the World Bank was to hold its final meeting with donor nation representatives to plan the implementation and financing of its Third Population and Family Health Project for Bangladesh. The report was written to directly influence officials involved in that meeting. Its charges may be summarized as follows:

1. There really is (or should be) no problem of over-population in Bangladesh; the entire "population problem" is a convenient myth used by the Bangladesh government with donor connivance to avoid needed socioeconomic reforms and redistribution which could provide an adequate living for all.
2. The family planning and population control program of the government of Bangladesh is coercive because of its use of financial payments to those being sterilized and to service providers. The piece of clothing provided to sterilization acceptors (a sari for a woman, a lungi for a man) is not surgical apparel for sterile purposes, as the government and donors state, but one more inducement.
3. The donors and the government show a callous disregard for the human rights of family planning clients. Conditions in clinics are deplorable, informed consent is ignored, and clients suffer unaided with numerous side-effects and health problems after sterilization.
4. The emphasis is on fertility control and the extra fees to be earned by fieldworkers for doing this work has tended to bias the whole health delivery effort away from improvements in maternal and child health, nutrition, and other urgently needed programs.
5. The major donors, especially A.I.D., the World Bank, and UNFPA, pay for the program and essentially dictate policy. It is under pressure from them that the government has made population "the number one priority" and effectively ignored other needs.

Both works confuse ideology with evidence. Consequently, the conclusions drawn by their authors do not accurately portray the realities of Bangladesh. Underneath their authoritive facade, these publications are little more than political tracts which express the biases of their respective authors. For example, *The Deadly Neo-Colonialism* condemned the Bangladesh program on the grounds that it was proceeding toward "the Chinese model." In contrast, *Food, Saris, and Sterilization* praised the Chinese approach, saying that Bangladesh should use that model instead. The Hartmann-Standing publication circulated widely among U.S. feminist groups, several of whom subsequently wrote to policy-makers in Washington repeating the charges and demanding or asking for explanations and changes. The O'Reilly publication circulated widely among U.S. right-to-lifers and natural family planning proponents, many of whom lobbied Congressmen and other policy-makers in Washington demanding that U.S. support to family planning in Bangladesh be discontinued or radically changed to favor only natural family planning. Eventually the Hartmann-Standing publication caught the attention of O'Reilly who used it to support conservative right-wing arguments in a subsequent publication of Human Life International titled, to provoke alarm, *USAID's Agenda of Fear* (O'Reilly 1987).

The Reality

Sterilization services are easily the most closely monitored and thoroughly studied component in the Bangladesh health and family planning program. The government of Bangladesh, donors, and various non-governmental organizations have invested a great amount of time and several millions of dollars on sterilization-related monitoring, research, and evaluation. Since 1980, there have been more than a dozen major sterilization-related research and evaluation efforts that focused solely or partly on issues of voluntarism. The U.S. government alone (through A.I.D.) has since 1983 funded approximately 20 quarterly sterilization surveys. As international attention focused on sterilization in Bangladesh, the number of studies and evaluations increased. Methodologies were developed and refined to measure the degree to which people chose sterilization voluntarily, their satisfaction with the procedure, and the effects of compensation payments on the sterilization decision-making process. Hundreds of other research studies and evaluations have focused on related aspects of family planning. In short, the Bangladesh family planning program is among the best studied in the world.

The remainder of this chapter will show that the critics' charges are not borne out by this extensive body of research. Conclusions from this research, and related research that addresses the critics' charges, are as follows:

1. The Bangladesh program is not coercive.
2. The decision of Bangladeshi men and women to undergo sterilization is a carefully considered, voluntary act, chosen from among several different methods of birth control. Exceptions are very rare and are becoming rarer as detailed knowledge about family planning becomes increasingly widespread.
3. Payments to clients, which are made to compensate them for costs incurred in the process of having and recovering from a tubectomy or vasectomy, help broaden contraceptive choice by providing access to sterilization for those who otherwise could not afford to use the method, or who would otherwise defer the operation until some later date (frequently after an unwanted pregnancy terminated by abortion or followed by the birth of an unwanted child).
4. The international donor agencies that contribute funding for the Bangladesh family planning program do not control it.
5. The population problem in Bangladesh is not a myth used to avoid needed reforms. Family planning is just one part of a broad range of development efforts undertaken by the government of Bangladesh and donor organizations, which, along with activities in agriculture, education, health, housing and energy, include such reform-directed activities as improving the status of women and stimulation of rural industry.

Sterilization

Much if not most of the turmoil over the Bangladesh program was invoked by the word "sterilization." A red flag goes up for many people when they hear the word—sterilization is immoral, illegal, or at least it is something which should not be encouraged. Some religions prohibit sterilization and some countries even have laws against it (Sai 1986:8). Even many Americans who believe that sterilization is a good birth control option whisper the word in hushed tones or they use a euphemism—as in "I'm going to get my tubes tied."

Nonetheless, sterilization is by far the most preferred form of birth control in many countries. Indeed, the world leader is the United States, where over 40 percent of married women of reproductive age are protected by tubal ligation or the vasectomy of their husbands (Ross, Hong and Huber 1985; Philliber and Philliber 1985). Sterilization now accounts for approximately one-third of all contraceptive practice in the world; over 100 million couples now use sterilization as their method for preventing unwanted births.

For women and men who have completed childbearing, there is technically no better method. For men, sterilization (vasectomy) is a very safe and simple out-patient procedure. Sterilization procedures for women (tubectomy or tubal ligation), while more complicated than vasectomy, are nevertheless also relatively safe and simple—especially compared with the risks of childbirth when it takes place at home attended by family members or traditional birth attendants untrained in sterile techniques and unable to handle serious complications (see also Hern's chapter in this volume, and Potts, Speidel, and Kessel 1978).

The demand for sterilization is steadily rising in developing countries. However, demand far exceeds the supply of services, which until recently were virtually nonexistent in the rural areas of many countries (Kessel and Mumford 1982). In some developing countries, sterilization is not part of the government's national family planning program, often because of religious opposition. In many other countries, it is provided by family planning programs only with a great number of restrictions—restrictions, in fact, that many Americans, women in particular, would consider an infringement of a basic human right. In Bangladesh, for example, primarily because of high infant mortality, regulations specify that no one may receive a sterilization through the national family planning program unless he or she already has at least two surviving children over the age of one.

The popularity of sterilization in many developing countries, especially among poor, rural people, is easy to understand. In the U.S. and most other developed countries, the prevalent pattern of marriage followed by a period of time when the couple does not want children results in high demand for temporary methods of .contraception. This desire for temporary contraceptive methods is augmented by the current pattern of intercourse and cohabitation before marriage. The desire to space children for health, economic, ease-of-childcare, and other reasons also contributes to Westerners' demand for temporary contraception. Circumstances are quite different in developing countries.

In many of these countries, women's welfare continues to depend on demonstrated fertility and women commonly become pregnant and produce a child as soon after marriage as possible. Many women are also subject to pressures to produce one, two, three, or more surviving sons. Under such circumstances, many woman are given little chance to space births, or to prevent births, until they have four, five, six, or more children. A one-time procedure that prevents all future pregnancies is very attractive to women who have already produced a large family.

This is true in Bangladesh, which is a very poor, conservative, predominantly Muslim society. Traditionally, young girls enter arranged marriages in their early teens and are expected to begin producing children immediately and remain in their homes, illiterate and in purdah (seclusion from men who are not relatives) or semi-purdah. Men hold power over women and want sons (Ahmed 1981; Chaudhury and Ahmed 1980; Ellickson 1975; Alauddin 1980; Schuoustra-van-Beukering 1975; Cain, et al. 1979). Daughters usually are not treated as well as sons, and are far more subject to abuse and neglect (Chen et al. 1981; Bairagi 1986). The legal restrictions that Bangladesh has placed on the provision of sterilization services reflect, at least partly, the considerable pressure on married women to produce at least two surviving sons. Son preference thus contributes to high infant mortality rates via neglect of female infants, and, so, to closely-spaced pregnancies that reduce maternal health (Hossain and Glass 1988; Aziz and Maloney 1985). Recent surveys suggest that Bangladeshis want an average of 3 to 4 children. Women need an average of about 5 live births to achieve this family size, given the very high infant mortality levels. Living circumstances are so severe for the majority of rural Bangladeshis, however, that few, men or women, want many more than this number.

Family Planning in Bangladesh

Family planning has become well known throughout Bangladesh. Over 90 percent of Bangladeshi adults now know about modern family planning. Although it is still not so widely or regularly used as in many other developing countries, about 30 percent of Bangladeshi couples of reproductive age now use some form of contraception, modern or traditional (Bangladesh Contraceptive Prevalence Survey, Mitra and Kamal 1985). (This contrasts, for example, with 65 percent in Thailand and 60 percent in Colombia. The comparable figure in the United States is about 70 percent [Ross, Hong and Huber 1985].)

The World Bank and the U.S. Agency for International Development (A.I.D.) are the major foreign donors that support the Bangladesh government's family planning program. A.I.D. began assisting family planning efforts in Bangladesh (formerly East Pakistan) in 1965 and was joined subsequently by the World Bank, support from which now considerably exceeds that from A.I.D. (Pillsbury, Kangas, and Margolis 1981). The UNFPA, European aid agencies, and many private donors also provide support to family planning in Bangladesh.

A full range of contraceptive methods is used in Bangladesh today. Many traditional methods (herbal, magical, religious, and other) are still widely used, often in combination with modern methods (Maloney, Aziz, and Sarkar 1980). All major modern methods are available and knowledge of family planning methods is nearly universal among adult Bangladeshis. Family planning is sanctioned by the Quran, which speaks of withdrawal (*azl*) and advises people to have no more children than they can provide for. Nearly all (over 95 percent) women of reproductive age report that they know about female sterilization and the oral pill and the majority also know about condoms and vasectomy. Pills and condoms are almost universally available through door-to-door delivery or in local pharmacies and shops. IUDs are provided in over 1500 locations. Other methods are also quite widely available (Mitra and Kamal 1985:89; Choudhury 1985:13).

Temporary methods of contraception, like the pill or condoms, however, require repeated contact with health and family planning workers. Cultural rules of purdah (and, in many areas of the countryside, real danger for unaccompanied women) prevent many women from leaving the immediate vicinity of their home. This means that contraceptives like pills and condoms, and follow-up for IUDs, must be provided on a door-to-door basis by family planning fieldworkers who must go out from clinics to the homes of individual clients. Health and family planning fieldworkers, however, are low-level civil servants. Like other such civil servants in Bangladesh, many regard their jobs as sinecures and it is difficult to motivate them to work and, especially, to make these home visits (Koblinsky et al. 1984). These cultural obstacles to the provision of family planning services are compounded by poor communication and trans-portation facilities, which makes the delivery of services of any kind very difficult. Most rural homes have neither electricity nor clean or running water, for example. Many roads wash away annually in the monsoon season when some 10 to 20 percent of the country is flooded and many villages are cut off from the outside for months at a time. In the home, potential storage areas for pills or condoms are often not safe from children, moisture, or insects.

Thus, it is not surprising that voluntary sterilization (also known as voluntary surgical contraception, or "VSC") has gradually become the leading method of contraception in Bangladesh. Sterilization was intro-duced almost 25 years ago on a pilot basis in 1966 when Bangladesh was still East Pakistan. Today about two-fifths of Bangladeshi couples who use some form of contraception have had a sterilization (38.5 percent in 1983).[2] Both male and female sterilization (vasectomy and tubectomy) are performed. Female sterilization is virtually all "interval sterilization" (i.e., not immediately postpartum), since nearly all births take place in the home. The oral pill is the second most common method, used by about one-fifth of contracepting Bangladeshis (17.2 percent in 1983) (Mitra and Kamal 1985). The IUD, condoms, and vaginal foams are also widely available throughout the country.

Sterilization services are provided by the Bangladesh government as part of its general family planning program, by the Bangladesh Association for Voluntary Sterilization (BAVS), by several other non-governmental (private and voluntary) organizations, and by private physicians. It is government policy that all sterilizations in Bangladesh are to be carried out on the basis of voluntary, informed consent. Sterilization services, except by private physicians, are provided free of charge.

Sterilization services are not targeted at poor, rural women, or at any other category of people. There is no policy to target information or services disproportionately to any one group; nor is there any evidence of bias on the basis of sex, age, religion, residence, or economic status. Rural areas are emphasized, for example, simply because over 85 percent of the people live there. As for the charge of targeting women, many more tubectomies were performed than vasectomies in the early 1980s, but vasectomy has gained popularity in recent years. In 1985, about 115 vasectomies were performed for every 100 tubectomies.

About 80 percent of Bangladeshis are Muslims and about 15 percent are Hindus (the remaining five percent are chiefly Christians or animists). Tubectomy rates among Hindu women have been somewhat higher than among Muslim women. Among Hindu men, however, vasectomy rates are considerably lower than among Muslim men. The precise reasons for these differences are not clear, but there is no evidence that any special efforts have been made to "target" either Hindu women or Muslim men—or any other religious or ethnic group (Quasem July-Sept. 1985, pp. 43, 46). There is no organized religious opposition to sterilization.

The Reimbursement/Compensation System

As in other South Asian countries, the government of Bangladesh has for many years (since 1965) made modest payments to facilitate and encourage the use of sterilization and also the IUD. As of 1985, when the events upon which this chapter focuses were taking place, A.I.D., as part of its overall support to family planning in Bangladesh, was reimbursing the Bangladesh government for certain costs related to the provision of voluntary sterilization services—including training, medical quality control, research, evaluation, and so on (Oot et al. 1986).

Among these costs were reimbursements for three types of compensation payments provided by the Bangladesh government to certain categories of persons. One is "client compensation." The sum of 175 takas (about $5.30, at the current rate of exchange) is given to men and women (clients) who undergo sterilization to reimburse them for out-of-pocket expenses and to compensate for foregone income or lost worktime. A second type is the "helpers' compensation." The sum of 45 takas (about $1.36) is given to a family planning worker or another person who accompanies a client to and from the health center and assists him or her while there, to compensate for this helper's costs and services. The third is a per-case payment to service providers (physicians receive 20 takas, or about 61 cents, and clinical assistants receive 12-15 takas, or about 36-45 cents).

The purpose of this compensation system is to neutralize financial barriers to the use of sterilization services. The "helper" compensation, for example, was instituted in view of the fact that most rural Bangladeshi women live in a state of purdah or semi-purdah and are culturally forbidden to leave their homes or move about in public freely. The presence of a "helper" makes culturally acceptable, and safer, the journey to the clinic, which often is many hours away from the woman's home by public transport. Also, many women who have a tubectomy are still breastfeeding and thus must take their youngest child with them and have someone to care for it during and after the surgery. Many women would not be able to overcome the prevailing cultural and logistical obstacles if they did not have a "helper" to accompany them to and from the clinic and care for their child during surgery.

Moreover, in this country where health facilities characteristically are rudimentary at best, sterilization is usually the first operation that a person has had. It may also be the first time that this person has even stepped inside a clinic or encountered Western medicine. For men as well as women this is often a frightening experience that requires moral support. Frightening, too, is the need to deal with strangers who, for illiterate villagers, stand far above them in the caste system. A person who approaches another whose position is higher feels most comfortable with an intermediary who can bridge the gap of rank and introduce a personal element into a process where impersonal relationships are threatening (see Cleland and Mauldin 1987:20 and Schuler et al. 1985). In addition, given the lingering false notion that vasectomy is a form of castration, many Bangladeshi men are nervous and apprehensive (just as are many American men) over the possibility that the operation may render them impotent. Thus, just as in the United States, albeit for a different set of reasons, both men and women who go to a hospital for surgery need someone to accompany them, so too do many Bangladeshi men. Recognizing this, the "helper" compensation was also made available for persons who accompany a vasectomy client, as well as a tubectomy client, to assure that this assistance will be available and to compensate the helper for his or her expenses.[3]

The Bangladesh government routinely compiles statistics on the number of procedures that have been done. As of 1985 when the attacks described above were mounted, the Bangladesh government then submitted these figures to the local United States Agency for International Development office (USAID/Dhaka) with a request for reimbursement. USAID/Dhaka has routinely scrutinized these figures in light of other data received from its monitoring and surveillance systems. When problems have arisen or where discrepancies existed, USAID/Dhaka has decreased proportionately the amount of its reimbursement and acted immediately to resolve the problem.

Safeguards, Monitoring, and Research on the Bangladesh Sterilization Program

The Bangladesh government has established clear policies and directives that all sterilization (like all family planning) must be voluntary. Procedures have been established to ensure that these policies are carried out throughout the country. These include: eligibility criteria, informed consent requirements, client screening and counseling, and monitoring systems. Where monitoring systems, general surveillance, or the press have raised questions that could not be answered by other sources, special research studies have been undertaken.

Eligibility Criteria

To be eligible for sterilization, a Bangladeshi must be in adequate physical condition to undergo surgery and must have at least two children, the youngest of which is at least one year old. The purpose of this is to reduce the possibility of post-sterilization complications and regret.

Informed Consent

All requestors are required to have a basic understanding of sterilization and its effects, including its permanency. Policies are designed to ensure that all requestors document their consent to the operation. A.I.D.-approved informed consent forms, which are consistent with those used in the United States, are filled out prior to surgery by nearly all people (98 to 99 percent) who undergo sterilization (Quasem 1985:26, Oot et al. 1986:24).

Client Counseling and Screening

Each person who requests sterilization goes through a two-part screening on arrival at the clinic. The first step is to determine that requestors meet the family size and informed consent requirements. The second step is medical screening. Requestors who do not meet the eligibility requirements are "rejected" and counseled to use some other method of family planning until such time as they may meet the requirements.

Monitoring Systems

Clearly, in any large national program deviations and problems can occur. The Bangladesh government and the donors know this and have therefore instituted several systems to monitor the effectiveness of the eligibility, informed consent, and screening requirements. The intent is not merely to minimize deviations, but also to detect and resolve potential problems before infringements occur. These monitoring systems have included:

- *The Family Planning Clinical Surveillance Team* (FPCST), formerly called the *Voluntary Sterilization Surveillance Team* (VSST). This is an international team (headed by the World Health Organization representative) that travels throughout Bangladesh inspecting clinics and identifying areas that need improvement. While the principal focus is on improving medical quality, the team also monitors counseling, screening, and informed consent practices to ensure that sterilization is being undergone on the basis of informed voluntary consent.
- *The Implementation, Monitoring, and Evaluation Division of the Planning Ministry.* The population section of this division is responsible for monitoring the national family planning program, and conducts on-site reviews of compliance with sterilization informed consent and reimbursement policies.
- *Quarterly surveys of BAVS services.* Internal auditors of BAVS, Bangladesh's largest non-governmental provider of sterilization services, have monitored use of informed consent forms and conducted periodic audits of clinic activity to verify clinic performance, service quality, and client satisfaction.
- *The Quarterly Evaluation of the National Sterilization Program.* This analysis was initiated (and paid for) by USAID/Dhaka as yet an additional verification that sterilization procedures were being performed in accord with U.S. government regulations. This analysis was based on a nationally-representative sample of male and female sterilization clients, as well as service providers in both public and private health facilities. Topics covered included monitoring of reimbursement payments, client characteristics, use of informed consent forms, and verification of reported performance. The evaluations were conducted (up through early 1988—see below on "The Denouement") by M.A. Quasem & Co., an independent, private-sector Bangladeshi firm.
- *Ongoing surveillance.* In addition to the formal systems above, government and donor agency staff have continuously monitored

the sterilization program through field trips and review of key service statistics, such as sterilization incidence, method mix, characteristics of people who adopt sterilization, requestor rejection rates and reasons, and referral patterns.

In addition, Bangladesh has an active, fairly free press which, like that in the United States, is eager to expose problems of many kinds, including occasional problems concerning sterilization.

These monitoring and surveillance systems have uncovered a few violations or potential violations of the government's voluntarism policy. The first of the now much-publicized problems arose in late summer 1983 when the army was assisting relief and health activities in the aftermath of massive flooding in the Mymensingh area. In the course of their efforts, army officials took it upon themselves to "help" family planning workers by using military ambulances to transport sterilization clients to clinics. When USAID/Dhaka and Ministry of Health and Family Planning officials learned of this, they rushed representatives to the site, investigated the situation, and halted it. The government in Dhaka promptly ordered the military to avoid all further such involvement with family planning.

A similar incident in which local officials from outside the family planning program also took it upon themselves to assist the national family planning goals occurred in certain parts of Bangladesh in late 1984 and early 1985. In this instance, local officials decided to require that women must have had a sterilization in order to receive free donor-provided food supplies. This situation occurred in the "Vulnerable Group Feeding" program which distributes food to needy Bangladeshis. It is managed centrally by the United Nation's World Food Programme but is administered in the rural areas by elected local officials called union council chairmen. Because supplies were not adequate to go to all in need, some means had to be devised to decide who should receive the food that was available. Some union chairmen, eager to assist the government in its family planning effort and independent of any discussion with superiors, decided to add to the requirements for receiving food that women getting the food must have been sterilized. Standard criteria of the Vulnerable Group Feeding program do not even require women to be users of family planning at all. Adding the sterilization requirement was clearly a violation of existing policy. Fortunately, there were no reports of ineligible, unwilling, or unprepared women getting sterilized in order to get the food, but the mere existence of such a prerequisite clearly violated World Food Programme, government, and donor policies prohibiting such inducements. Once the Ministry of Health and Family Planning became aware of the situation, swift corrective action was taken including a formal government directive banning any linking of such welfare benefits to the condition of family planning acceptance.

To help verify that the sterilization requirement had been more of a potential than an actual problem, and that corrective actions were effective, USAID/Dhaka added questions to the Quarterly Evaluation of the National Sterilization Program to determine if sterilization clients were promised or actually given anything other than the program-approved compensation and surgical garments. None of the sterilization clients interviewed in connection with the 1985 second-quarter evaluation reported receiving food or any other unapproved items (Quasem 1986), and no new incidents have been reported. The World Food Programme subsequently added questions to verify that sterilization is not being used or perceived as an eligibility requirement for this feeding program to the monitoring guidelines used by its field officers. There have been no similar problems since.

Special Research

In addition to ongoing monitoring, by 1985 a large number of studies of the sterilization decision-making process, client satisfaction, the role of compensation, and improving services had been undertaken, many in response to concern about the compensation system. These studies included:

- *The Female Sterilization Follow-Up Study of 1984.* This was a survey of 920 women who had received sterilization in 1984 at one of nine BAVS clinics in different parts of Bangladesh. Findings of this carefully executed study describe the sterilization decision-making process, motivation for having the operation, and sources of sterilization-related information (Mitra and Associates 1985).
- *A Ministry of Health and Population Control Client Satisfaction Survey.* This study of a nationally-representative sample of 2,377 men and women who were sterilized at government and NGO facilities during 1983 and 1984 was funded by the Swedish International Development Authority (SIDA), an influential donor in Bangladesh and one highly concerned about moral and human rights issues related to the sterilization compensation system, and was undertaken by P&M, a private Bangladeshi firm. Findings provide data on topics including clients' information sources, characteristics, and levels of satisfaction (unpublished P&M study reported in Newton 1985).
- *The Population Development and Evaluation Unit [of the Planning Commission of the Bangladesh Government] Evaluation of the Sterilization Program* (Miah and Rahman 1987). This study surveyed 807 men

and women who had had sterilizations at government and NGO facilities to determine if they were pleased with sterilization and why they were or were not.

- *The 1983 Contraceptive Prevalence Study*. This carefully executed survey, which was the largest survey ever undertaken in Bangladesh, involved approximately 20,000 household interviews conducted between October 1983 and January 1984 (Mitra and Kamal 1985).
- *The SIDA-Sponsored In-Depth Case Study of Health and Family Planning in Two Villages in Comilla Division*. This was a "user-perspective" study in which three female (and feminist-oriented) researchers lived in a rural community and employed anthropological techniques to evaluate the government program from the viewpoint of the consumer. This study provides insightful descriptions of village attitudes toward family planning and the government family planning program, including sterilization services (Akhter, Banu, and Feldman, 1983.)

Additional studies at that time included:

- *Female Acceptor Focus Group Study* (M. Alauddin and Sorcar 1984).
- *Volunteerism and Satisfaction: A Focus Group Study of Sterilization and IUD Acceptors* (F. Alauddin, Sorcar, and Rahman 1988).
- *The Voluntary Surgical Sterilization Team "Before and After" Survey*.
- *The PIACT Referral Fee Study* (Choudhury 1985).
- *The PIACT Study on Motivational Factors that Determine the Non-Use of Contraceptives* (Choudhury et al. 1985).
- *The ICDDRB Follow-Up Survey of Sterilization Acceptors* (Bhatia 1979).

The large amount of research activity in this area was itself a positive sign that the Bangladesh government seriously intended to develop a more effective yet still voluntary family planning program. Most importantly, results showed that the existing family planning program was not coercive. The compensation payments were generally having their intended effect—they have made it possible for people who want no more children to achieve that goal fairly soon after they make that decision.

The Sterilization Decision-Making Process

The catalyst to begin "seriously thinking" about sterilization is usually a pregnancy or birth of a child. For nearly all couples, this is a third or subsequent birth that results in a family of 2 sons and 1 (or more) daughter(s). Sterilization is used almost solely by couples who have a minimum of 3 children. Couples who choose sterilization have, on average, about 4 living children at the time they undergo the procedure. Given the high infant mortality rates in Bangladesh, such couples are likely to have experienced 5 or more live births.

Couples whose children are still so young as to be at high risk of dying, or couples who are apprehensive about going to a strange place (the clinic) and having surgery, may prefer initially to try pills or condoms. It is common, however, for rural illiterate women who have never taken any medicine in their lives to use the pill irregularly and thus find themselves with an unwanted pregnancy. It is also an unwanted pregnancy such as this that makes many couples decide to have a sterilization. The study by Alauddin and Sorcar (1986) found that about 25 percent of sterilization clients interviewed had previously had an abortion. Such women see sterilization as a way to avoid another abortion.

Once a woman enters the "serious consideration phase," she almost always discusses her interest in becoming sterilized with two or more relatives or friends—her husband and women who have already had the operation, as well as with mothers- and sisters-in-law. Of women interviewed in the BAVS survey, 98 percent discussed the idea with their husbands, 77 percent with already-sterilized women, 26 percent with mothers-in-law, and 24 percent with sisters-in-law (Mitra and Associates 1985:35-38, 68-70).

A woman gets specific sterilization-related information from already-sterilized friends, neighbors, or relatives, or from family planning field-workers. In many villages, almost every adult knows who has been sterilized and which women have used pills (Akhter, Banu and Feldman 1983:133). The vast majority of women who decide to have a sterilization report that other sterilized women were their first source of specific sterilization-related information and, along with family planning field-workers and husbands, furnished the most information. This includes information about the nature of the operation, when and where it is available, who can provide help in getting to the clinic, and the fact that money is available to defray some or all of the costs (Choudhury 1985:13). Ready access to satisfied clients appears to allow Bangladeshis to refine and confirm the information on which they are basing a sterilization decision (see the next section).

The compensation payment does not appear to be an important influence on the decision as to whether or not to get sterilized. Rather, it is important because it enables individuals to have the operation relatively soon after making the decision to become sterilized (Newton 1985). This finding emerges both from survey research and qualitative research. Farida Akhter, Fazila Banu, and Shelley Feldman, who conducted

the ethnographic village study in Comilla Division, concluded, for
example:

> . . . findings among our sample population do not confirm the notion
> that [the compensation payments], in and of themselves, are a motivational
> mechanism, nor did they appear to act significantly differently among
> different classes of people participating in the Government's programme.
> Most clients agreed that the money they received from the Government's
> programme would ensure that the operation and required stay at the
> Family Welfare Center would not cost an individual out-of-pocket expenses
> . . . [but] would be used to cover the costs incurred in transportation to
> the Center and food for the client, her children, and other persons
> accompanying her (Akhter, Banu, and Feldman 1983:78).

This study also found that some women were forced to borrow money
from others to cover the costs of their stay at the health center. (Clients
do not receive the compensation payment until ready to leave the center
after surgery.) Borrowing this money, they found, sometimes required
paying interest or incurring other obligations. In addition, the costs of
having water and food, neither of which are provided at the health
center, purchased and brought from the local bazaar, exceeded the actual
reimbursement. The study concluded that "In short, in almost all cases,
there is no actual economic benefit gained" from the compensation
payment, that it "was not a major attraction for accepting sterilization,"
and that it "does not act to independently bring people for sterilizations"
(Akhter, Banu, Feldman 1983:78-79). These conclusions are especially
significant, coming as they do from a team at least one of whom has
been highly critical of the government family planning program.

For the vast majority of clients, the decision to have a sterilization
appears to be made prior to arrival at the clinic. When a Bangladeshi
woman arrives at a clinic, she has already crossed most of the cultural,
psychological, and logistical obstacles to sterilization and the purpose
of her visit is to be sterilized, not to collect additional information about
sterilization or other birth control options.

After a woman decides to have the operation, there is still a de facto
waiting period. Once she conveys her decision to a family planning
fieldworker, with whom a surgery date is scheduled, several days or
even weeks usually elapse while logistical arrangements (including
arrangements for childcare and being accompanied to the clinic) are
finalized. This waiting period appears to present adequate opportunity
for reconsideration. An average[4] of 7 to 12 months lapse between the
time a woman begins considering sterilization as a birth control option
to the time when she actually has the operation. Some women report

having considered sterilization for as long as four years (Alauddin and Sorcar 1986).

Client Satisfaction

The circumstances of Bangladeshi couples, the time that they take to decide on sterilization, the range of alternatives they have to choose among, and the extensive social interaction that is part of the decision to sterilize make it clear why men and women who have had the operation say, almost without exception (96 to 98 percent), that they are satisfied with their choice. Why? Clients know before the operation its effect and permanence (Mitra and Associates 1985:123) and have a good idea how it will affect their lives (see Miah and Rahman 1987).

Large numbers of men and women who have chosen sterilization recommend it to friends, neighbors, and relatives. Almost half of the tubectomy clients in the Female Follow-Up Survey said they had already recommended the operation within a few weeks after having had the procedure, and 96 percent said that they intended to do so (Mitra and Associates 1985:122-125). And 76 percent of vasectomy clients and 83 percent of tubectomy clients in the P&M Client Satisfaction Survey sample said they had recommended sterilization to others while 90 percent said that they intended to do so (P&M 1985:128, 336, 338, 392, in Newton 1985).

Why do so many Bangladeshis voluntarily choose sterilization? The basic reason is the same as in other countries—they do not want any more children. Why? Mostly to avoid the economic burden of a child that they can ill afford. Many Bangladeshi women also say that they choose sterilization because another pregnancy would be hard on their health, which in many cases is already poor. *No one*, of all the people who were interviewed in all of the studies cited above, said that he or she was compelled or deceived into getting sterilized. The compensation payment certainly was not the major reason. For example, 96.2 percent of the women interviewed in the BAVS survey did not even mention the reimbursement at all. Of the small (3.8) percent who did, none said that it was the primary reason (Mitra and Associates 1985: 70-72).

There is a high level of community support for sterilization. Over 90 percent of sterilized men and women polled in the national P&M survey said that their family and friends approved their decision to have the operation. This finding also suggests that the act of having a sterilization is one which people discuss quite freely, at least among family and friends. Opposition from local religious leaders was common in the late 1970s and even early 1980s but is now greatly diminished. In fact, many religious leaders or their wives are now reported to have undergone sterilization (Alauddin and Sorcar 1986). The extensive public social interaction which surrounds sterilization provides an atmosphere in which coercion, if there were any, would become widely discussed and denounced.

Few people express dissatisfaction with the procedure or regret over having had it. Only 1.6 percent of respondents in the BAVS survey, for example, said they were dissatisfied in some way. The tiny minority who felt this way did so either because a pregnancy occurred anyway, because of health reasons that were unrelated to the operation (e.g., chronic abdominal pain that a woman hoped would concurrently be cured by the sterilization), or (for some women) because the physician who performed the operation was a man. Side-effects—real, imagined, or falsely attributed—are another source of dissatisfaction, but rarely lead people to regret having had the operation. Some who said they regretted the operation went on to express general regret at being poor and not able to afford a large family. No one reported having been pressured or deceived into having the operation.

Actual regret is not common and appears to occur, as one might expect, among couples who later experience the death of a child (Cleland and Mauldin 1987:ix). Requests to have a sterilization reversed (recanalization) clearly indicate regret. The Bangladesh government offers recanalization with expenses paid, and two or three Bangladeshi surgeons are able to perform the reversal operation. To date there have not been many requests for reversal. The low levels of dissatisfaction and regret further indicate that sterilization decisions are being made in a well-informed and voluntary manner (Newton 1985:13). Levels of regret in Bangladesh appear no higher than, and actually may be lower than in many other countries, including the U.S. (Philliber and Philliber 1985:14–15, Henshaw and Singh 1986).

The "Incentive" Question

The data reviewed in this chapter make it plain that Bangladeshis who choose to use sterilization do so voluntarily, typically after long and careful consideration, without coercion, and with their informed consent (also see M. Alauddin and Sorcar 1984, F. Alauddin and Sorcar 1986, Cleland and Mauldin 1987, and Alauddin, Sorcar and Rahman 1988). They do so because it makes sense to them, as it would to most of us if we shared their circumstances.

While the monitoring and research described above showed that Bangladeshis were not being coerced into sterilization against their will, a somewhat separate question persisted as to whether the payments constituted "incentives." Many donors as well as developing country governments believe that the use of incentives to encourage family planning is appropriate and desirable in developing countries that face problems of rapid population growth—provided that the incentives are not large enough to motivate people to do something they otherwise would not want to do. The U.S. Congress has approved the use of incentives in A.I.D. family planning programs, within limitations. However, it prohibits the use of financial incentives that lead clients to favor one method of contraception over another.

This prohibition provided one more angle of attack for the critics of the Bangladesh sterilization program. Did the compensation payments in Bangladesh constitute financial incentives? Did they motivate people to choose sterilization over other methods of contraception? The critics said "Yes."

They argued that the compensation payments were more than the actual costs and resulted in Bangladeshis becoming sterilized "for the money." This was especially true, many critics argued, in the case of "unemployed housewives" who, "because they have no job outside the home should not be compensated for lost work time."[5] One A.I.D. official (a Reagan administration political appointee) who was critical of the program, but who had never set foot in Bangladesh, asserted: "With the extra money a housewife like this gets, she can add a new wing to the family house."

Critics also argued that the garment (sari or lungi) provided for clients to wear during surgery was yet another incentive—luring, it was implied, innocent victims to undergo this awful thing. On this topic, the same Reagan appointee commented: "I bet lots of those women just see sterilization as a chance to get a new party dress."

Given the ongoing concerns, in late 1985 both A.I.D. and the World Bank launched further studies to answer definitively the questions of whether sterilization in Bangladesh was truly voluntary and whether the compensation payments led Bangladeshis to choose sterilization over other alternatives. The A.I.D.-sponsored study (Pillsbury and Knowles 1986) concluded that reimbursement payments were approximately equal to the average costs and wage losses incurred and that the primary incentive to choose sterilization was not money but to end childbearing and prevent unwanted pregnancies.

The analysis also concluded, however, that the government's use of an *average* cost reimbursement system made it possible for a minority of individuals to realize a small monetary gain (equivalent to a fraction of the $5.30 in the case of a patient or $1.35 in the case of a helper). Just as insurance companies in the U.S. and elsewhere frequently reimburse patients and providers for surgical procedures on the basis of average costs, so, too, the Bangladesh government had concluded that is is

necessary, for administrative and monitoring purposes, to compensate
on the basis of average costs, rather than attempt to reimburse actual
costs on an individual basis, especially given the millions of individuals
involved. (This is the same principle that the U.S. government and many
private firms follow, for example, in establishing the per diem rates that
apply to all employees who visit a given city, regardless of the precise
expenditures of the individual visitor.)

Some clinics in Bangladesh (those of BAVS) have in the past attempted
to reimburse actual costs on an individual basis. However, if the government were to try reimbursing sterilization clients on an individual
basis, it would create not only an administrative nightmare but greatly
increase opportunities for corruption. It is also likely that this would
result in compensation levels higher than the current levels (as occurred
when BAVS attempted to reimburse on an individual basis). An average
cost reimbursement scheme encourages patients and their helpers to
limit their actual expenses.

Patients who live close to a health facility or who make a quick post-
surgical recovery may find that the compensation payment leaves them
with a few extra takas. These are likely to be used to buy a fish or a
few eggs to supplement the daily diet of rice and lentils. The cavalier
suggestion that the few Bangladeshis who are over-reimbursed can use
their "profits" to "put an extra wing on the house" is absurd. Patients
who live farther from a health facility or who experience post-surgical
complications, of course, find that their compensation payment does not
cover all their costs.

The above analyses also revealed that the garment (sari or lungi)
given to a patient during surgery does *not* constitute an incentive to
use sterilization, contrary to critics' assertions. These garments are
provided to minimize the risk of infection, as is a patient gown in any
hospital. The Bangladeshi patient, however, keeps the garment and is
encouraged to wear it home post-surgically, because the everyday sari
or lungi is often used for many unhygenic purposes (including wiping
a child after he or she defecates).[6] In fact, the saris and lungis given to
sterilization patients are not highly valued. Many rural Bangladeshis
criticize the government for giving them such a poor quality garment
and do not wear it after surgery. Some give it away to a poorer person,
or use it only as a liner for a mattress or as a fabric to put under an
infant to catch its feces (Pillsbury and Knowles 1986, Kotalova 1984:28).
This is a far cry from being "a new party dress."

Enter the U.S. Congress

The 1985 attacks on the donors for their support of the sterilization
program in Bangladesh made these donors, especially A.I.D., extremely

worried that during the spring 1986 Congressional season conservative Congressmen might be pressured to terminate all support for family planning in Bangladesh. Throughout this time, the then chief administrator of A.I.D., M. Peter McPherson, was embroiled in trying negotiate continued U.S. support for UNFPA activities globally—in the face of continuing assaults by opponents of international family planning who sought to terminate all U.S. assistance to UNFPA on the grounds that it was contributing to abortion in China. This endeavor consumed more of McPherson's time than any other single issue he had to confront as A.I.D. administrator (Crane and Finkle 1989:37). The attacks on A.I.D. for its support of sterilization in Bangladesh mounted in intensity at roughly the same time.

In the end, however, the Bangladesh family planning program never became the issue that was predicted. Senator Jesse Helms, Representative Jack Kemp, and others made hostile inquiries, but this whole subject faded that spring when Congressional debate became dominated by the question of whether or not to grant then-President Reagan his desired $100 million in aid to the Nicaraguan Contras. The crisis for Bangladesh family planning support, it seemed, had passed, and U.S. reimbursement of the sterilization payments continued.

Many right-to-lifers, however, remained committed to reducing support for international family planning, or shifting it over to only "natural family planning." U.S. feminists' criticism of sterilization and such methods as Norplant or Depo-Provera continued to provide fuel for the right. Hartman and Standing's *Food, Saris, and Sterilization* became grist for Human Life International's publication *USAID's Agenda of Fear* (O'Reilly 1987), which further asserted that A.I.D. was violating human rights in Bangladesh and sought to spark Congressional investigation. Donor agencies remained concerned.

The Denouement

Results of the long-awaited World Bank-sponsored study, *Study of Compensation Payments and Family Planning in Bangladesh*, finally became available in early 1988. It was funded by the European "like-minded" donors—chiefly governments of northern European countries which, unlike A.I.D., had not funded the compensation payments, disliked their use, and threatened to withdraw all financial support from the Bank's family planning project unless it conducted a thorough and definitive study of the payments. The study took two years to complete, and was based on eight separate studies and surveys, the results of which were summarized and analyzed by two of the world's leading family planning experts, John Cleland and Parker Mauldin (1987).

"We have found no evidence of coercion," concluded this extensive and authoritative study (Cleland and Mauldin 1987:50). The report elaborated:

Sterilization clients know beforehand that the procedure represents a permanent end of childbearing. . . . Sterilization decisions in Bangladesh are firmly founded not only on the principle of informed consent but also on the principle of prior thought about sterilization, including discussions with a wide range of people such as friends and relatives (who have no vested interest) and with individuals who have undergone sterilization. . . . The decision of an individual to be sterilized is primarily the result of a feeling that their family size is as large as they want (70%) or is already too large (30%). Among respondents in the clinic-based survey, 41% said they had not wanted their last pregnancy (Cleland and Mauldin 1987:13).

"There is no evidence to suggest that sterilizations are performed on people who do not want to limit their family size," concluded Cleland and Mauldin (p. 15). "Family size limitation is the dominant motive for seeking sterilization" (p. 15).

These resoundingly positive conclusions were followed, however, with a statement that became the guillotine for A.I.D. financing of the compensation system. This was that, for a minority of clients, "the prospect of a small cash balance after expenses have been met is probably an incentive" (p. 15). Despite hundreds of pages of documentation that the payments were *not coercive*, the authors' use of the single word "incentive" led the newly-appointed chief administrator of A.I.D., Alan Woods, a former press aide to Richard Nixon and Assistant Secretary for Defense, to stop U.S. reimbursement for the Bangladesh compensation payments in early 1988. Woods reportedly had little patience for the whole issue anyway and did not want to alienate Congressional supporters from whom he needed backing on other issues that he considered more important.

The Bangladesh government considers the compensation payments sufficiently important that it now allocates funds of its own to cover the costs of clients and providers. However, it has terminated the helper payments, a situation that some researchers feared would cause many family planning workers to remain in their offices rather than go out to village homes and escort clients back and forth to health centers. The USAID-funded quarterly evaluations of the sterilization program also have stopped. Many observers of the program fear that A.I.D., without its financial involvement in the compensation system, will not be able to continue its systematic monitoring and surveillance, and encouragement to the Bangladesh government in these matters—attention which was previously so crucial in assuring that sterilization remained voluntary. In the end, the politics of family planning in the U.S. may have worsened rather than improved the circumstances of a people and country most in need.

Bangladesh ranks near the bottom of the International Human Suffering Index (Camp and Speidel 1987). It is one of the world's poorest yet most densely populated nations with about 100 million largely malnourished and illiterate people crowded into an area only the size of Wisconsin. With few exceptions, one can stand anywhere in rural Bangladesh and be surrounded by human settlements. Eighty-five percent of Bangladeshis live in rural areas; there 30 to 40 percent of the population is unemployed or underemployed, 50 percent are landless, and landlessness is increasing. Sixty percent of the rural population gets less than 85 percent of the calories required for minimum subsistence. Competition for scarce resources is fierce (Harris 1985; Cain and Mozumder 1980; Jannuzi and Peach 1978).

According to some analysts, rural unemployment is likely to attain staggering proportions, straining and breaking down the traditional rural safety net. In the last decade, poverty, misery, and, in many communities, crime and violence, have actually increased (Robinson 1985). There is the specter of a famine of unthinkable magnitude produced by a simultaneous decline in food availability and loss of exchange entitlements (Jansen 1986). In the meantime, many peasants who have been squeezed off productive land have moved onto marginal, previously uninhabited, low-lying lands from which many are periodically swept into the sea by tidal floods. In May 1985, for example, at the same time that the anti-sterilization protests were being levied in Washington, D.C., at least 10,000 Bangladeshis perished in a cyclone that struck the low-lying Gangetic island of Urirchar.

Bangladesh's population is growing rapidly and most analysts agree that unless this growth can be slowed, all other development efforts will be in vain. Indeed, in Bangladesh, the reality is that the country will be lucky if population growth does not effectively block all development efforts. Under the best scenario, Bangladesh must ultimately live with double the number of people who now live there. What is at issue is whether Bangladesh's population will merely double or will grow to three or four times its present size.[7] Cessation or serious interruption of the family planning program would be disastrous for the future of the entire country as well as for the hundreds of thousands of individuals who are family planning clients—and for whom risks of pregnancy, especially *unwanted* pregnancy, are great. Estimates are that more than half a million women in developing countries die every year in pregnancy or childbirth. The proportion of women who die due to pregnancy-related causes in Bangladesh is among the highest in the world (Lettenmaier et al. 1988; Potts, Speidel and Kessel 1978). Under present circumstances, it appears prudent that the Bangladesh government continues to compensate people who want to use sterilization, despite family planning and reproductive rights battles being waged in the United States.

Obviously, family planning alone can never be the solution to Bangladesh's problems.[8] The Bangladesh government and dozens of international donors are putting enormous amounts of money and technical assistance into other development activities, including rural development, agriculture, education, and health services. But development activities that might improve women's status and lead to a transition from high to replacement-level fertility are even more difficult to carry out on any wide-scale basis than it is to provide reliable, high quality family planning services.

Women's opportunities to become educated or to improve their status vis-a-vis men remain sorely constrained (Abdullah and Zeidenstein 1982; M. Islam 1985; R. Islam 1981; S. Islam 1982; Lindenbaum 1981). Some analysts (e.g., Chen 1983) see indications of greater opportunity for some women. However, the pauperization of women is increasing in many rural areas (Westergaard 1983). A recent study ranked the status of women in 99 countries, using measures of health, education, employment, and social equality (Camp 1988). The women of Bangladesh were at the bottom of the list. Bangladesh is one of the few countries in the world where the life expectancy of women (only 49) is lower than that of men—a major cause of early female death being pregnancy, childbirth, and abortion to terminate unwanted pregnancies. The health of women and children will also remain poor so long as high parity and short birth intervals continue to prevail.

Continued improvements in the Bangladesh family planning program, as in anything else, depend on well-reasoned criticism based on sound observations.[9] Ideologues, however, tend to confuse belief with evidence and to substitute their own interests for those of the people whom they claim to serve. Continued ill-informed attack might easily deny the Bangladeshis who are most in need of what feminist critics, and most Americans in general, consider an essential human right, namely the right to knowledge, information, and services for family planning. This would deny to many Bangladeshis what may be the most fundamental of all human rights—the right to exert some effective control over one's own life.

Notes

1. See Crane and Finkle (1989) for an excellent analysis of the campaign waged by the New Right, including their supporters in the White House and State Department, to eliminate all U.S. support to international family planning and population activities in 1981—efforts that culminated in 1985 to focus on China and then Bangladesh. See also Johnson and Reich (1986) "The New Politics of Natural Family Planning."

2. Although sterilization is the most common method of family planning in Bangladesh, less than nine percent of all Bangladeshi couples of reproductive age have had (either the husband or wife) the procedure. This is a very small percentage in comparison to 41 percent in the United States or even to other developing countries such as Colombia and Panama (about 30 percent) or neighboring Thailand (about 28 percent).

The popularity of sterilization in Bangladesh climbed from the early 1980s through November 1984, but has since declined (as measured by the number of new acceptors each year). The reasons for the decline are not understood. The decline may be: (1) evidence of "saturation"—that most high parity couples who firmly desire to terminate childbearing and who have access to a family planning clinic have already had a sterilization operation; (2) further evidence that the compensation is not enough to induce people to have the operation if they do not want it; and/or (3) due to low morale among family planning workers.

3. The terms "referral agent" and "referral fee" have also been used for the person who accompanies a client to the clinic, but the terms "helper" and "helper's fee" more accurately reflect the nature of the task. A.I.D. has never reimbursed the Bangladesh government for referrals, only for operations performed.

4. This "average" is, in fact, a median.

5. A.I.D. and the Bangladesh government had deliberated long and hard over the question of compensation to women clients. In the end, and consistent with the views of Bangladeshi women activists, they concluded that women who were "housewives" were not, in fact, unemployed (see Wallace et al. 1987, S. Islam 1985, Loutfi 1985), and that it would be discriminatory to refuse them compensation. (The total work time loss compensation for women is 75 takas, or about $2.25; the total work time loss compensation for men is 117 takas, or about $3.50.) In addition to child care, labor-intensive food preparation, gathering cow-dung for fuel, fetching water, harrowing the fields, hauling heavy loads, and other physically demanding work, women spend a great deal of time processing rice and other food products that would be factory-processed and readily available for purchase in other countries. The loss of a woman's labor, even for the two days when she is absent for surgery and the 5 to 9 days following the surgery when she is to refrain from abdominal strain and contamination of the incision, involves significant costs for the average low-income

family. Either the husband must stay home from work, or relatives and neighbors must be imposed upon, which incurs a debt that must be repaid somehow.

6. Saris are commonly used in rural Bangladesh to clean eating utensils, hands, dirty children, eyes (which may have conjunctivitis), or to blow a nose or wipe the unwashed anus of a child (Stanton and Clements 1986:486, Kotalova 1984).

7. Julian Simon and others may contend that there is no population problem in the world today, since difficulties caused by imbalances between populations and resources will be overcome within 30 to 80 years (Simon 1981). The cost in human suffering of waiting out those years, however, might well be catastrophic in a country like Bangladesh.

8. The "natural family planning" advocated by right-wing critics is certainly not the answer (see Johnson and Reich 1986). Natural family planning methods depend on some combination of detection of cervical mucus, determination of basal body temperature, and periodic sexual abstinence. These are not feasible for many Bangladeshi couples and are associated with significant failure rates even in countries like the United States. The argument that such methods are hazard-free is groundless. In reality, the use of natural family planning significantly increases the risk of unwanted pregnancy and its associated health hazards (see Hern's chapter in this volume; Hughes 1988:9).

9. See Tinker (1982) "Feminist Values: Ethnocentric or Universal?"

References Cited

Abdullah, T.A. and S.A. Zeidenstein. 1982. Village Women of Bangladesh: Prospects for Change. New York: Pergamon Press.

Ahmed, N.R. 1981. Family Size and Sex Preferences among Women in Rural Bangladesh. Studies in Family Planning 12:100–109.

Akhter, Farida, Fazila Banu, and Shelley Feldman. 1983. An Assessment of the Government's Health and Family Planning Programme: A Case Study of Daudkandi Thana and North Mohammadpur and Charcharua Villages in Bangladesh. Dhaka: Swedish International Development Authority. ·

Alauddin, Fateema and Nihar Ranjan Sorcor. 1986. Motivation and Decision-Making in Voluntary Sterilization: A Focus Group Study Conducted December 1985–February 1986. Dhaka: Family Development Services and Research.

Alauddin, Fateema, Nihar Ranjan Sorcar, and Azizur Rahman. 1988. Voluntarism and Satisfaction: A Focus Group Study of Sterilization and IUD Acceptors. Dhaka: Family Development Services and Research.

Alauddin, Mohammad. 1980. Socio-Economic Determinants of Fertility in Bangladesh: A Review. Dacca: University of Dacca, Institute of Social Welfare and Research.

Alauddin, Mohammad, and Nihar Ranjan Sorcar. 1984. Focus Group Discussions with Sterilized Women in Bangladesh. Mimeo. Dhaka: Family Development Services and Research.

Aziz, K.M. Ashraful and Clarence Maloney. 1985. Life Stages, Gender and Fertility in Bangladesh. Dacca: International Centre for Diarrheal Disease Research, Bangladesh.

Bairagi, Radheshyam. 1986. Seasonal Food Shortage and Female Children in Rural Bangladesh. American Journal of Clinical Nutrition 43:330–332.

Bhatia, S. et al. 1979. A Follow-up Survey of Sterilization Acceptors in the Modified Contraceptive Distribution Project. Dhaka: International Centre for Diarrheal Disease Research, Bangladesh, Scientific Report. No. 19.

Bangladesh Association for Voluntary Sterilization (BAVS). 1984. Skills Needed by An Effective Counselor. Dhaka.

Cain, M.T., et al. 1979. Class, Patriarchy, and Women's Work in Bangladesh. Population and Development Review 5:405–438.

Cain, Mead, and A.B.M. Khorshed Alam Mozumder. 1980. Labor Market Structure, Child Employment, and Reproductive Behavior in Rural South Asia. Working Paper No. 56, Center for Policy Studies, The Population Council, New York.

Camp, Sharon, ed. 1988. Poor, Powerless, and Pregnant: Country Rankings of the Status of Women. Washington, D.C.: Population Crisis Committee.

Camp, Sharon and J. Joseph Speidel, eds. 1987. The International Human Suffering Index. Washington D.C.: Population Crisis Committee.

Chaudhury, R.H. and N.R. Ahmed. 1980. Female Status in Bangladesh. Dhaka: Bangladesh Institute of Development Studies.

Chen, L.C., E. Huq, S. D'Souza. 1981. Sex Bias in the Family Allocation of Food and Health Care in Rural Bangladesh. Population and Development Review 7:55–70.

Chen, M.A. 1983. A Quiet Revolution: Women in Transition in Rural Bangladesh. Cambridge: Schenkman Publishing Co.

Choudhury, Abu Yusuf. 1985. Report on a Study of the Referral Fee System in the Population Control Program. Dhaka: Program for the Introduction and Adaptation of Contraceptive Technology.

Choudhury, Abu Yusuf, Safiqur Rahman Choudhuri, Md. Najmul Huq, and Atiqur Rahman Khan. 1985. Motivational Factors That Determine the Non-use of Contraceptives. Dhaka: Program for the Introduction and Adaptation of Contraceptive Technology.

Cleland, John and W. Parker Mauldin. 1987. Study of Compensation Payments and Family Planning in Bangladesh. Dhaka: World Bank and NIPORT.

Congressional Record. 1986. House of Representatives: Abortion Battle Shifts to AID for Family Planning. U.S. Congress, Proceedings and Debates of the 99th Congress, Vol. 132, No. 11. (Feb. 6). Containing reprint of article by Toner, Robin, Abortion Battle Shifts to AID for Family Planning. New York Times (Feb. 5, 1986).

Crane, Barbara B., and Jason L. Finkle. 1989. The United States, China, and the United Nations Population Fund. Population and Development Review 15: 23–59.

Edmonds, Scott W., Donald H. Minkler, Barbara L.K. Pillsbury, and Michael H. Bernhart. 1985. The Performance of the Association for Voluntary Sterilization in Developing Countries, 1982-1985. Washington, D.C.: International Science and Technology Institute.

Ellickson, Jean. 1975. Rural Women. In Women for Women, pp. 81–89. Dhaka: University Press.

Harris, M. 1985. Inheritance Patterns and Land Fragmentation in a Bangladesh Village. Bangladesh Advisory Research Council Consultancy Report.

Hartmann, Betsy, and Hilary Standing. 1985. Food, Saris, and Sterilization: Population Control in Bangladesh. London: Bangladesh International Action Group.

Hasan, Yousuf and Marjorie Koblinsky. 1985. Motivating Workers to Work: Part I. Dhaka: International Centre for Diarrhoeal Disease Research, Bangladesh.

Henshaw, Stanley K. and Susheela Singh. 1986. Sterilization Regret Among U.S. Couples. Family Planning Perspectives 18(5):238–240.

Hossain, M. Moshaddeque and Roger I. Glass. 1988. Parental Son Preference in Seeking Medical Care for Children Less Than Five Years of Age in a Rural Community in Bangladesh. American Journal of Public Health 78(10):1349–1350.

Hughes, Janice. 1988. Natural Family Planning: Very Risky Business. Conscience 9:7–12.

Huq, Jahanara, Roushan Jahan, and Hamida Akhtar Begum, eds. 1985. Women and Health. Report of the End-Decade National Conference on Women and Health Organized by Women for Women and Concerned Women for Family Planning. Dhaka: Women for Women.

Islam, Mahmuda. 1985. Women, Health, and Culture. Dhaka: Women for Women.

Islam, R. 1981. Women, Work and Wages in Rural Bangladesh. Journal of Social Studies 11:56–69.

Islam, Shamima. 1985. Invisible Labour Force: Women in Poverty in Bangladesh. Dhaka: BRAC Printers.

Islam, Shamina, ed. 1982. Exploring the Other Half: Field Research with Rural Women in Bangladesh. Dhaka: Women for Women.

Jannuzi, F.T. and J.T. Peach. 1978 (?). Report on the Hierarchy of Interests in Land in Bangladesh. Dhaka: United States Agency for International Development.

Jansen, Eirik G. 1986 Rural Bangladesh: Competition for Scarce Resources. Oxford: Oxford University Press.

Johnson, Jeanette, and Julie Reich. 1986. The New Politics of Natural Family Planning. International Family Planning Perspectives 12:132–143.

Kessel, Elton, and Stephen Mumford. 1982. Potential Demand for Voluntary Female Sterilization in the 1980s: The Compelling Need for a Nonsurgical Method. Fertility and Sterility 37(6):725–732.

Koblinsky, Marjorie, Ruth Simmons, James Phillips, and Md. Yunus. 1984. Barriers to Implementing an Effective National MCH-FP Program. Dhaka: International Centre for Diarrhoeal Disease Research, Bangladesh.

Koblinsky, M.A., et al. 1986. Daily and Monthly Work Routines of the Government Family Planning Worker: The Family Welfare Assistant (FWA). Dhaka: International Centre for Diarrheal Disease Research, Bangladesh, MCH-FP Extension Project Working Paper No. 9.

Kotalova, Jitka. 1984. Personal and Domestic Hygiene in Rural Bangladesh. Dhaka: Swedish Development Cooperation Office and Swedish Council for Research in the Humanities and Social Sciences.

Lettenmaier, Cheryl, Laurie Liskin, Cathleen Church, and John A. Harris. 1988. Mothers' Lives Matter: Maternal Health in the Community. Population Reports, Issues in World Health. Series L, No. 7. Baltimore: Johns Hopkins University.

Lindenbaum, S. 1981. Implications for Women of Changing Marriage Transactions in Bangladesh. Studies in Family Planning 12:394–401.

Loutfi, Martha F. 1985. Rural Women: Unequal Partners in Development. Geneva: International Labour Office.

Maloney, Clarence, K.M. Ashraful Aziz, and Profulla C. Sarkar. 1980. Beliefs and Fertility in Bangladesh. Rajshahi: Rajshahi University, Institute of Bangladesh Studies.

Miah, J.A. and M.B. Rahman. 1987. Assessment of Satisfaction of the Sterilization Acceptors. Dhaka: Planning Commission, Population Development and Evaluation Unit.

Mitra, S.N., and G.M. Kamal. 1985. Bangladesh Contraceptive Prevalence Survey—1983. Dhaka: Mitra and Associates.

Mitra, S.N., M.F. Karim and B. Khuda. 1986. Female Sterilization Follow-up Study—1984. Dhaka: Mitra and Associates and Bangladesh Association for Voluntary Sterilizaton.

Newton, Gary. 1985. A Report on the Voluntarism of Sterilization Services in Bangladesh. Dhaka: Association for Voluntary Surgical Contraception. (Unpublished Report, December 8).

Oot, David, Sallie Craig Huber, John Knodel, and Alan Margolis. 1986. An Overal Evaluation of the USAID/Bangladesh Family Planning Services Project (388-0050): Key Issues and Future Assistance. Arlington, VA: International Science and Technology Institute.

O'Reilly, William M. 1985. The Deadly Neo-Colonialism: Report on Population Control in Bangladesh. Washington D.C.: Human Life International.

———. 1987. USAID's Agenda of Fear. Washington D.C.: Human Life International.

Philliber, Susan G. and William W. Philliber. 1985. Social and Psychological Perspectives on Voluntary Sterilization: A Review. Studies in Family Planning 16(1):1–29.

Pillsbury, Barbara L.K., Lenni W. Kangas, and Alan J. Margolis. 1981. U.S. Assistance to The Family Planning and Population Program in Bangladesh, 1972–1980. Washington D.C. and Dacca: Agency for International Development.

Pillsbury, Barbara L.K. and James C. Knowles. 1986. Is Sterilization Voluntary in Bangladesh? A Study of Reimbursement Levels for Sterilization in Bangladesh. Washington D.C.: International Science and Technology Institute.

Potts, Malcolm J., J. Joseph Speidel, and Elton Kessel. 1978. Relative Risks of Various Means of Fertility Control. In Risks, Benefits, and Controversies in Fertility Control. J. Sciarra, G. Zatuchni, and J.J. Speidel, eds. Pp. 28–51. New York: Harper and Row.

Quasem, M.A., and Co. 1985. Report on the Evaluation of the Voluntary Sterilization Program for January–March Quarter 1985. Dhaka.

Quasem, M.A., and Co. 1986. Report on the Evaluation of the Voluntary Sterilization Program for July–September Quarter 1985. Dhaka.

Rahman, M., D. Huber, and J. Chakrovorty. 1987. A Follow-up Survey of Sterilization Acceptors in Matlab, Bangladesh. Dhaka: International Centre for Diarrheal Disease Research, Bangladesh, Working Paper No. 9.

Reichley, A. James. 1984. Religion and Political Realignment. Brookings Review 3:29-34.

Robinson, Warren C. 1985. Some Reflections on Recent Attacks on the Population Program in Bangladesh. University Park, Pennsylvania: Institute for Policy Research and Evaluation. Mimeo.

Ross, John A., Sawon Hong, and Douglas H. Huber. 1985. Voluntary Sterilization: An International Fact Book. New York: Association for Voluntary Sterilization.

Sai, Fred T. 1986. Some Ethical Issues in Family Planning. Paper presented at conference, Ethical Issues in Reproductive Health: Religious Perspectives. Washington D.C.: Catholics for Free Choice.

Schuoustra-van-Beukering, E.J. 1975. Sketch of the Daily Life of a Bengali Village Woman. Plural Societies 6:51–66.

Schuler, Sidney, E. Noel McIntosh, Melvyn Goldstein, and Badri Raj Pande. 1985. Barriers to Effective Family Planning in Nepal. Studies in Family Planning 169(5):260–270.

Simon, Julian. 1981. The Ultimate Resource. Princeton: Princeton University Press.

Stanton, Bonita and John D. Clements. 1986. Soiled Saris: A Vector of Disease Transmission. Transactions of the Royal Society of Tropical Medicine and Hygiene 80:485–488.

Tinker, Irene. 1982. Feminist Values: Ethnocentric or Universal? Washington, D.C.: Equity Policy Center.

Wallace, Ben J., Rosie Mujid Ahsan, Shahnaz Huq Hussain, and Ekramul Ahsan. 1987. The Invisible Resource: Women and Work in Rural Bangladesh. Boulder: Westview Press.

Westergaard, K. 1983. Pauperization and Rural Women in Bangladesh: A Case Study. Comilla: Bangladesh Academy for Rural Development.

World Federation of Health Agencies for the Advancement of Voluntary Surgical Contraception. 1984. Ensuring Informed Choice for Voluntary Surgical Contraception: Guidelines for Counseling and for Informed Consent. New York.

11

The Politics of AIDS, Condoms, and Heterosexual Relations in Africa: Recent Evidence from the Local Print Media

Caroline Bledsoe

The presence of AIDS (Acquired Immunodeficiency Syndrome) in Africa has triggered enormous international concern. Although AIDS may have relatively little long term impact on the overall population growth in Africa because of continued high birth rates (Bongaarts 1988, and van de Walle & Palloni 1987), the disease is bound to have severe impacts on mortality. It will also create massive economic problems stemming from losses of productivity, training, and diversion of funds from development to crisis health care.

Mortality rates and economic problems, however, may prove less serious in the long term than social devastation. Already the AIDS epidemic has begun to exacerbate existing social and political tensions, leading to panic reactions that scapegoat vulnerable groups. Since considerable attention has been devoted already to prostitution as the primary means of HIV (Human Immunodeficiency Virus) spread in Africa, this paper turns to the epidemic's impact on potentially stable heterosexual relations, particularly from women's perspectives. By identifying some of the assumptions that comprise similar cultural themes in these countries, it examines some bellweather trends in people's emerging responses to policy injunctions to limit partners and use condoms. I draw policy conclusions for three topics:

- the fate of children whose mothers die from AIDS
- threats to female education in the wake of the AIDS epidemic

• cultural interpretations of condoms and the likelihood of condom acceptance

In setting about this task, I point out that people do not necessarily respond to policy directives in ways outsiders might predict. African peoples set their own agendas for change in culturally specific ways (see Ajayi 1969 and Peel 1983). As such, they appear to be interpreting official AIDS advice through their own cultural categories. They are also attempting to avoid the constraints posed both by AIDS dangers and policy directives. Such facts suggest that "unintended consequences" of policy actually follow logically, given certain underlying cultural premises and principles of social dynamics.

I am interested in technology and how it travels and takes root, or is rejected, in places where it did not begin. As social scientists, we easily identify differences between our own and other people's cultural beliefs when examining rituals or artifacts that are very different from our own. Ironically, we tend to overlook the strength of different indigenous beliefs when they are manifested in technologies such as condoms that outwardly resemble our own. One reason why a transplanted technology may be rejected is that it may be reinterpreted with a meaning more familiar to the new context. This paper asks how condoms, once placed in the African context, take on meanings that their outside promoters may not fully appreciate.

Condoms have worked well in other parts of the world. But in Africa they pose large problems. They obstruct fertility, a key African value. More subtly, they become symbols of social distance that most women do not want to put between themselves and their male partners. Finally, they intrude into the delicate process of developing conjugal relations— a process that must eventually include childbearing. Although I examine a problem of medical origin, therefore, I try to step behind the cultural lens of the peoples who are being advised to adopt what to many are offensive prophylactic technologies. I conclude, however, that despite the difficulties that condoms pose, persistent efforts to introduce them as part of AIDS education packages in secondary schools make sense according to some important cultural logic.

Data and Methods

The information used here stems from two sources. The first is prior research on the complexities of domestic and conjugal relationships among the Kpelle people of Liberia (e.g., 1980) and the Mende of Sierra Leone (in press, b). Whenever possible, though, I prefer to let people themselves speak in the cultural categories they are assembling to make sense of a frightening disease that is disrupting the very fibre of their most basic social relations. For the other source, therefore, I took an unconventional approach, on the gamble that it could yield surprising insights. I searched for recent quotes from Africans themselves on the subject of AIDS—quotes that reflect current attitudes toward AIDS, condoms, and policy injunctions. One source of such quotes is the research of *Projet Connaisida*, which began working in 1985 in Zaire on attitudes about AIDS and factors that expose women to risk. But primarily I use local African newspapers and journals, a source of data rich with cultural opinions and beliefs. My research assistant searched through some African newspapers from the last two years that Northwestern University Library has collected, particularly those from Central and Eastern Africa. He produced a pile of fascinating material, ranging from reports of local conferences to news items and letters to the editor. He avoided articles that appeared to have been reprinted from international wire services, unless they contained quotes, preferably direct, from Africans.

Analysts accustomed to quantitative evidence may well raise the issue of sampling problems. In terms of content, items taken from newspapers are rarely routine or typical. If they were, they would not be newsworthy. Yet as Goffman (1974:14–15) points out for his own extensive use of newspaper material for sociological analysis, the very fact that people have selected these incidents as worthy of public discussion and elaboration bespeaks their cultural significance. The quotes I have found mirror the social world, commenting on its assumptions, predicaments, and possibilities for reconstrual. By highlighting, as few other sources could, the evolving dynamics of sexual mores and evolving conjugal dilemmas that debates over AIDS have spawned, they allow us to extrapolate policy implications that are sensitive both to local life as well as to trends much broader in scope.

A second problem of content concerns the views expressed in newspapers. Even within the publications, of course, there was by no means a uniformity of opinion. Particularly letters to the editor varied widely in the extent to which the authors felt AIDS was a problem and, if so, in what measures should be taken to stem its spread. I try, therefore, to give some indication of variance, even though I may use only one quote.

Third, although most of the publications used here are not the main government newspapers that are obliged to report the party line, virtually all African newspapers are subject to government scrutiny and possible dismantling for stepping too far out of bounds. I also use several quotes from a Catholic newspaper, *The National Mirror* of Zambia. These political and religious factors would suggest that while biases undoubtedly appear in the reporting, these newspapers would tend, if anything, to suppress discussion or to slant coverage and views in conservative directions. Despite these pressures, the reporting is remarkably frank, a fact of particular significance in the face of criticism that African governments have received in the last few years for failing to acknowledge the reality of AIDS in their countries.

Besides problems of content, a problem of volume inevitably arises as well. Although I have selected certain quotes, it may appear that these are the only ones to be found. These quotes, however, were actually selected out of a large number of similar quotations. The ones used here were simply the best or the most explicit.

A final question concerns cultural heterogeneity. The quotes come from several countries: principally from central and eastern Africa (Zaire, Zambia, Tanzania, and Uganda) but also from West Africa (Nigeria and Sierra Leone). The idea of constructing a unitary cultural perspective from such disparate ethnic groups and countries seems indefensible. Nonetheless, certain themes appeared with striking consistency: problems for fertility that condoms pose, the association of condoms with promiscuity, economic pressures that induce women to contract lovers, polygamous tendencies among men, school girls' vulnerability, and so on. Consequently, I allowed these to dominate the analyses and to shape its conclusions concerning the impact of AIDS on relationships between men and women and the policy speculations for the issues of female education, condom adoption, and welfare of AIDS orphans.

Contemporary Pressures on Women That Increase AIDS Risks

To understand local people's responses to AIDS and to policy measures that are being taken to stem its spread, we need to begin by looking at the cultural notions of heterosexual relations that underlie all this, particularly two fundamental premises involving marriage and fertility.

1. Marriage, as a process, frequently entails testing out relations among potential partners.
2. At some point fertility becomes central to the marriage process, and the partner who cannot or will not have children is soon abandoned.

Two additional factors complicate these processes. The first is an increasing trend to educate young women. This prolongs the marriage process, thereby opening the potential for relations with more sexual partners. The second is growing economic pressure that contemporary women, including older school girls, find difficult to overcome without employing multi-partner sexual strategies.

Marriage

African women in their childbearing years spend relatively little time outside of conjugal relationships. Parents and family elders exert considerable pressure on young women to marry early and to remarry quickly upon divorce or widowhood. Yet African marriage is rarely a single event in time. More typically, it is a process that extends over a period of months or even years (see, for example, Evans-Pritchard 1951; Comaroff and Roberts 1977; Aryee and Gaisie 1979:287; Brandon and Bledsoe 1988; Bledsoe in press, b), as partners and their families work cautiously toward more stable conjugal relationships. At some point in the process, cohabitation and sexual relations begin, and children may be born. But these events do not necessarily coincide with, or follow predictably from, marriage rituals or economic transfers.

Because conjugal relationships can be developed gradually, a girl—sometimes with her family's implicit permission—may test out potential relationships with several young men before establishing a more permanent one. Older women in more established relationships may also contract sexual relationships with outside men, to keep alternatives open in case their current relationships become unsatisfactory. Obviously, the line between conjugal testing and actual prostitution can be very thin. Young women who cannot make ends meet by soliciting support from one partner may take on more partners on ever-more short-term arrangements. Whether we call this promiscuity, as many local people insist, or conjugal testing is less important than the realization that many women sustain sexual relations with several partners, either simultaneously or in sequence. (Following local practice, however, I will use the terms "husband" and "wife" when appropriate, to refer to partners whose relationship has become relatively stable.)

One of the most important factors underlying the marriage process is economics. Despite other sentiments influencing heterosexual relations such as affection, sexual desire, and the possibility of engendering children, most women depend on economic contributions from men. Without these contributions toward day-to-day expenses—contributions usually contingent on sexual favours—economic difficulties can undermine the solvency of women caught between decreasing opportunities to farm and an increasingly monetized cash economy, as Hilts (1988:29) points out for Uganda:

> The young women arrive in the city from the village, are unable to find
> work and so turn to the simplest means available to gain some money

and security. They seek men with means. The older men, who have jobs and often are married, find they can carry on such affairs with relative ease. . . . Many have accepted, if not approved, the habit among married and single men of moving from affair to affair.

These pressures threaten to intensify as national economic conditions deteriorate, and as cash, petrol, and food grow more scarce. Many women take up trade and other businesses in the informal sector. But even these women often it necessary to strike up "outside" or short-term relationships to tide themselves and their children over. Economic hardship particularly in the city frequently forces some women to become prostitutes. In the words of a Zambian reporter:

Sad stories are usually narrated by these girls who stand outside hotels when they are interviewed. A certain lady . . . said that "The reason why I do this is because I have two children, no husband, and so what else is there for me to do. I don't enjoy it but I have got no alternative" (*National Mirror*, Aug. 8, 1987).

Although actual prostitution is the exceptional case, sustaining an exclusive relationship with one man is not necessarily a woman's best economic strategy nowadays. Because of increasing economic hardship, even women with stable partners encounter pressure to find outside lovers, as a Sierra Leonean woman told me:

People are anxious to have this material wealth, and they can't get this money unless they go to their boyfriends [for help].

Fertility

Fertility remains a paramount value in Africa, and few areas have undergone anything resembling a fertility transition. Women can be divorced and men humiliated for not producing children. Adults want children for farm and household labor and for future support, and they hope some of their children will raise the family's status in the political world through formal schooling and urban employment. Within the contemporary climate of economic and political uncertainty in most African countries, moreover, children are valued as links to powerful patrons who can help their clients circumvent cumbersome bureaucratic channels to obtain jobs and money. Fertility is also important for women who seek to balance power vis-a-vis their co-wives. Even in co-wife relationships that commence amicably, a subfertile woman begins to realize that at best she is laboring in vain and at worst for the betterment of her rival's children.

Because of the value placed on fertility, women need children to build stable ties to men and their resource networks, to obtain money, clothes, and medical expenses (see also Frank & McNicoll 1987 and Guyer 1988). But high fertility can also backfire: hard times make children expensive if the father loses interest in them or cannot support them. Thus, although in theory fathers should pay most of their children's costs of schooling, medical treatment, and clothes, mothers often end up doing this. Young women who have not yet built up their trading businesses face have an especially difficult time supporting young children.

Just as sustaining several conjugal options necessitates multi-partner strategies, pressures to achieve high fertility motivate some women to conduct sexual relations with several partners. A woman who cannot conceive with her husband may turn secretly to an outside lover, or simply leave her husband and begin a relationship with another man. On the other hand, many women turn to outside men for monetary help in return for their sexual favours because they already have many children. Others find it increasingly advantageous to bear children by different men in order to gain access to several different resource networks. For Nigeria, Guyer (1988) shows that by contrast to *lineal* fertility theories, which stress the longterm returns to be gained from mature children, increasing economic instability is pressuring women to establish immediate *lateral* links with different men and their resource networks.

Children are at the heart of these lateral strategies. A woman can press her demands on a man with far greater leverage if she has a child by him, whether or not they call their relationship a marriage. The more networks to which a woman can create ties with her children, the more resources she can call upon, a strategy that Guyer calls "polyandrous motherhood." Children give solidity to old relationships without fore-closing new ones; marriage, in fact, becomes almost incidental to a woman's reproductive career. "The child is the key; without it there is no basis to claim anything beyond the moment of the relationship"(Guyer 1988:6).

Schooling

Although pressures for fertility remain on the whole, one large group of fertile women in Africa do *not* want to get pregnant: school girls. It may seem implausible to argue that schooling would pressure young women to contract sexual relationships. But school girls from non-elite families, especially, face severe pressure. Family elders recognize that the longer a girl remains in school, the more likely she may earn a good wage and become an elite urban man's wife. Yet they hesitate to spend money on her schooling, fearing she will get pregnant early and render their investments useless. Ironically, parental reluctance itself often makes this outcome a self-fulfilling prophecy: many secondary (and even some primary) school girls who badly want to continue their schooling become pregnant and drop out of school because they had to provide sexual favours in exchange for school fee money from older men, some of them highly placed politicians or senior civil servants (Bledsoe, in press, b). A writer in the *Zambian National Mirror's* "Women's Corner" complained that:

> The big men in Zmabia [sic] have also contributed [to the immorality in this country]. . . . These men who are often referred to as "sugar daddies" old enough to be fathers also go about for young girls and win their hearts by buying them presents and giving them a lot of Kwacha (Aug. 8, 1987).

Although parents sometimes send their daughters to expensive boarding schools to protect them from "sugar daddies," their efforts are easily undermined, as a letter to Uganda's *New Vision* deplored:

> Big men, traders, drivers to name but a few, used to go to nearby schools to steal [seduce] girls and spoil them. Good characters were spoilt and went for the worst. Gatekeepers of girls' boarding schools gained through bribery given to set free these girls to be taken by these men. . . . Special hire men were in business by transporting men and women to nearby lodges . . . (Aug. 19, 1988).

In some cases, parents themselves obtain assistance for their daughter's schooling from a man who helps pay her school expenses, and treat this as a preliminary marriage payment. But although many men view school fees as an investment toward obtaining a prestigious educated wife, others are married already and are committed to legal monogamy, which educated urbanites hold out as the mark of advancement. Although public outrage at such affairs is loud, private sentiment may support the liaison of a girl whose school career is in jeopardy. The editor of a Freetown newspaper column entitled "Women's Corner" responded thus to a girl whose school career was at risk:

> If you had a boyfriend who is prepared to help you he could see you through school. My advice is that you first of all look around for a relative of yours who is willing to help and if that fails then you get a man to help you. He might have to marry you before he takes the chance lest you slip away. I wish you good luck (*New Shaft*, Nov. 1, 1985).

In any event, because no one man is likely to help them consistently, some schoolgirls who need support turn to different partners and try, often by abortion, to avoid pregnancy long enough to complete their schooling. This observation tends to undermine a precept that is central to contemporary demographic transition theory—that educated women have lower fertility because they are educated. In the West African context, achieved educational levels tend to be a function of fertility— young women who manage to avoid pregnancy through birth control, abortion or infertility achieve higher levels of education than women who do not. Although some young women are taken out of school to marry and begin childbearing, many more must drop out because they got pregnant.

Finally, the prevalence of abortion among schoolgirls lends abundant testimony to the statement that schoolgirls have every desire to avoid pregnancy. Abortions comprise a rising major medical problem and a leading cause of death among young women in Africa (e.g., Kulin 1988). In some hospitals, almost half of the demands on scarce blood supplies are taken up by emergency transfusions for young women who have hemorrhaged trying to abort (Cherlin & Riley 1986). A Nigerian study found that 51 percent of maternal deaths at Lagos University Teaching Hospital stemmed from abortion complications (Akingba 1977). Of particular note for present purposes, most abortions appear to be performed on single, adolescent women in urban areas: very often teenaged schoolgirls (Frank 1985, Cherlin & Riley 1986, Caldwell & Caldwell 1988).

The Effects of Socioeconomic Pressures on AIDS Risks

Multiple partner strategies, despite their advantages in the deeping economic crisis, obviously take on new meaning in the light of the AIDS epidemic (see also Schoepf, in press). One might believe that the AIDS crisis should make women change their sexual behaviors. They might ask for financial help from their extended families rather than turning to outside sexual partners. But *Projet Connaisida* studies have found that poor families are increasingly unable to provide such help (Schoepf et al. 1988:217). When poor women must choose between immediate economic crisis in their households versus the remote possibility of contracting a dimly understood disease, the choice is easy. As *Projet Connaisida* research has found, "AIDS has now transformed what appeared to be a survival strategy into a death strategy" (Schoepf et al. 1988:217).

For schoolgirls as well, the AIDS crisis has sharpened the dangers in advancing their educations that heretofore entailed what now seem like relatively minor risks of pregnancy and school dropout. In response to these new threats, public AIDS education campaigns increasingly target their warnings toward schoolgirls, as a *Zambia Daily Mail* (May 2, 1988) article noted:

> . . . the adolescent category from which school pupils emerge as a higher-risk subcategory, needs to be a serious target for sex education.

Similarly, in Uganda, a District Administrator urged immediate government sponsorship for AIDS education campaigns, arguing that:

> Emphasis . . . should be put on the school age group, who are enticed to do what they should not by the sometimes infected well-to-do people through financial awards (*New Vision*, Sept. 22, 1988).

The Impact of AIDS on Relations Between Men and Women

Intensifying Suspicions

The main effect of the AIDS crisis on stable partner relationships appears to be that it deepens suspicions—previously a cause of much conjugal anguish, but one that has intensified enormously. Even relatives and casual friends retreat if suspicions of AIDS are whispered. In one of his weekly columns for the *Times of Zambia* (April 14, 1987), Mr. Kapelwa Musonda (a pen name) shows that because the AIDS hysteria has distorted people's usual common sense reactions, behavior that formerly was taken as routine can now be construed as evidence of AIDS:

> In such an atmosphere of uncertainty about the spread of the disease, one cannot afford to disappear from friends for unextended period [sic], become unhealthy or lose weight without incurring the suspicion that one has AIDS.

The main element of suspicion between spouses that arises in the AIDS crisis is promiscuity. If an individual tests positive for HIV, the association with promiscuity is almost inevitable, as columnist Musonda wrote in a passage displaying immensely elegant logic:

> Rumours and false alarming stories abound about who has it [AIDS], who might have it, who should certainly have it and well, if he or she doesn't have it, then it doesn't exist (*Times of Zambia*, April 14, 1987).

This association between AIDS and promiscuity usually leads to severe conjugal disruption, as a Ugandan counselor for AIDS victims related:

> . . . in most cases there are accusations. If one partner falls sick, the other says, "You have brought this disease" (Watson 1988:34).

Some consider such persons guilty of conduct so reprehensible that God is using AIDS as a weapon for divine punishment. One Christian writer in Nigeria, in fact, argued that God would protect the innocent spouse from contracting the disease, but would use AIDS to single out the guilty one:

> If after the observance of these elementary-like but divine rules by some while some break them, only the unfaithful partner would suffer any consequence of AIDS. The faithful partner would be mysteriously immunised by God the Almighty who is always very fair in his judgments, no matter how many time the innocent partner might have connections with the unfaithful partner-victim of AIDS (*New Nigerian*, March 9, 1987).

Men's and women's mutual suspicions of promiscuity are exacerbated by the realization that AIDS can be a lethal retaliatory weapon in the hands of vindictive spouses or jilted lovers. In stunning examples, embellished though they may be, Kapelwa Musonda (*Times of Zambia*, April 14, 1987) shows how AIDS has entered this cultural repertoire. I quote one example here:

> [A Lusaka man divorced his wife] after ten years of marriage on the grounds that she was unable to bear her husband any children. Instead, he married another woman who had claimed to have produced a child with him while he was still married to his first wife. It would appear things didn't work out as he had anticipated in his second marriage. He was unable to father another child and consequently, doubts and frustration about his manliness crept in and he began to feel he had been tricked into the new marriage. He slowly began to drift back to his old wife.
> In the meantime, the old wife, who had been very disappointed at being abandoned began to flirt around possibly in an attempt to prove to herself that she was still good enough for other men and she was in fact in demand. In the process she contracted AIDS and she was certified to be HIV positive. When one evening her old husband called on her and made some overtures, she literally dragged him into the bedroom. [She later reported:] "I never forgave that man for what he did to me. I was so depressed that I almost committed suicide. Now I have got him. You are talking to a woman who has committed a perfect murder. . . ."

Blaming Women

Whereas people acknowledge that HIV can be carried and spread by both males and females, it is striking how often media stories identify women as most at fault for spreading the disease to their partners.[1] For example, an advertisement placed in the *National Mirror* (Nov. 1, 1986) by a national Zambian organization called "The Fight Against the Spread of Aids" advised:

Avoid AIDS. Take Time to Know Her.

Similarly, accusations of using AIDS for witchcraft, an increasing theme, often single out women as witches, as in the following Ugandan case:

. . . when a man became infected, . . . his wife . . . worried that when the man died, the traditional healer would declare the cause of death to be witchcraft, not AIDS (Hilts 1988:30).

Accusations of immoral female behavior apply especially to alleged sexual crimes, as interviews with Zambian villagers revealed:

"Most people think AIDS is just the modern word for *amakombela*," said one man. It is believed *amakombela* is caught from women who have aborted or miscarried and have not undergone the traditional cleansing ceremony (*National Mirror*, May 14, 1988).

Perhaps because men's sexual affairs are generally overlooked while women are expected to restrict themselves to one partner, women's alleged promiscuity invites particular notice and provokes malicious gossip. Even if a woman contracted HIV from her husband, people still appear to assume that she was probably secretly promiscuous, as *Projet Connaisida* research found:

When men are infected, their wives are suspected of infidelity; when women are infected, they are assumed to have had multiple partners (Schoepf MS:5).

A married woman in Zaire described the stigma that women with AIDS incur, no matter how innocent they were:

Society rejects you. When you die you will not even be missed because you have died of a shameful disease. They will say that this woman has strayed. They will not see that maybe she has remained faithful while her husband has strayed. Given the status of women in most of our

African societies AIDS is doubly stigmatizing for women . . . (Schoepf, in press, p. 14).

Another of *Projet Connaisida*'s examples—a doctor whose two wives were blamed for promiscuity after they died of AIDS—shows how widespread such attitudes are even among educated people. A neighbor reported that the doctor himself

> . . . is still well and though he might be a healthy carrier people suspect the women of infidelity (Schoepf, in press, p. 11).

Local Responses to Policy Advice on AIDS Prevention

Recent Policy Measures

Government measures to combat the AIDS epidemic have been varied. In Kenya and Ethiopia, government officers periodically round up prostitutes in nightclubs and boarding houses (*Prize Africa*, Oct., 1986). In Uganda, President Yoweri Museveni opened a recent international seminar in Uganda on the Rights of the Child by suggesting that criminal charges should be brought against adults who seduce young people into illegitimate sexual activity with no intention of marrying them (*New Vision*, Nov. 24, 1988). He also warned that charges of assault and battery would be brought against AIDS victims who intentionally spread the disease, and that prostitutes and adulterers should receive corporal punishment (*New Vision*, Dec. 2, 1988).

Two of the more moderate measures that bear most relevance to my present purposes are the following admonitions: (1) limit sexual partners, preferably sticking to one partner, and (2) use condoms when engaging in sex outside marriage or with new partners—as a means to avoid AIDS or keep from spreading it. The Ugandan government best summed up both pieces of advice:

> "Love carefully": limit your partners, know them, and when in doubt, use a condom (Watson 1988).

For present purposes, I set aside three crucial issues—whether condoms are really safe, how much they cost, and how accessible they are. I simply note that condoms are technological devices—albeit ones that originated in the West—that allow people to follow policy advice, if they choose. Condom usage is advocated most particularly by World Health Organization, and is supported by growing numbers of other international agencies that are scrambling to subsidize and distribute condoms in Africa.

Condoms were created in the West for two primary reasons: to prevent the spread of sexually transmitted disease and to prevent pregnancy— especially pregnancy by a partner with whom one should not be engaged sexually. The recent experience of the outside world, at least before the AIDS crisis, has largely been that of distributing condoms to decrease pregnancies. For this purpose, condoms have worked moderately well in other parts of the world, especially places such as Japan and Thailand. In Africa, on the other hand, the primary purpose of condom distribution has become the prevention of the spread of a lethal sexually-transmitted disease. Preventing pregnancies is not generally a function that Africans who adopt condoms appear to want—with a few important exceptions, as we will see.

Individuals' Responses

If articles in local papers can be believed, some urbanites have indeed begun to use condoms. Campaigns to promote the use of condoms appear to have made the most impact where intensive efforts are exerted. In Kenya, nurse Elizabeth Ngugi is rapidly becoming famous for her work with Nairobi prostitutes, convincing up to 90 percent of one group to use them at least occasionally (Hilts 1988, 30). But limiting partners and using condoms are not easy resolutions to carry out consistently, as an East African woman pointed out:

> . . . neither abstinence nor total fidelity amongst married couples is a serious proposition in the real world in which adult men and women live . . . (*Weekly Review*, May 29, 1987).

Zaire's *Projet Connaisida* reports that among married women who had been counseled, most husbands flatly refused to use condoms or denied that there were AIDS risks to be concerned with, when their wives asked them to use condoms. Only one third of the husbands agreed to use them in principle. Actual practice was not discovered (Schoepf et al. MS:22).

Indirect evidence from newspapers also suggest that some urbanites have also begun to limit their partners. One major problem that obstructs compliance with this advice, however, is power imbalances between partners. Whereas AIDS information campaigns assume that individuals have complete control over their sexual lives, "stick to one partner" slogans may be irrelevant to those with little money or social status to refuse sexual demands. Unlike using other birth control prophylactics, using condoms requires the consent of both partners. This creates a particular problem for women, because they are usually subordinate in sexual relationships and hesitate to endanger economic support from men, as the Tanzanian *Daily News* (Dec. 1, 1988) suggested:

> Failure among some women to restrain from indiscriminate sexual habits, is mainly attributed to financial constraints . . . , according to some interviewees.

Power imbalances surface in other ways. One report suggested that if the woman gets sick and the man does not, the man is likely to evict her (Watson 1988:34). By contrast, in a case wherein the husband got sick, the wife remained, although she "left the marriage bed" (Hilts 1988:30).

Another obstacle to national policy efforts is that people may size up their options quite differently from how policy makers intend. Particularly if changing behavior involves great difficulty or economic loss, people tend to look for psychological loopholes. Denial is one of these: despite warnings, people can deny that the threat applies to them. In effect, they may change their behaviors in ways that appear to comply with the spirit of the advice when, from a Western medical standpoint, their behavior presents as much risk as before. For example, since weight loss is known to be a sign of AIDS, some men take only plump women as sexual partners. Other people, believing foreigners to be the primary source of AIDS, avoid them as sexual partners. Or, because HIV is reported to affect wealthy men and prostitutes, impecunious younger men may deny the dangers of their affairs with casual girlfriends. (See Schoepf, in press, for some examples of these tendencies.)

Besides psychological loopholes, many people look for epidemiological ones. For example, public education campaigns about AIDS have spurred some men not to cut down their sexual partners but to turn away from high risk groups such as prostitutes, and toward low risk pools. Whereas choosing plump partners may not represent the most medically sound strategies, therefore, considerable newspaper evidence of a new strategy has emerged that makes disturbingly good sense: older men have redoubled their attentions to schoolgirls, who represent the largest pool of unattached young women in urban areas. *Projet Connaisida* workers report that older businessmen who seek very young partners in order to avoid AIDS "can be observed parked at schoolyard gates waiting for girls to emerge" (Schoepf, in press, p. 12). Of course, in minimizing their own risks, these men raise those of young women, as Ugandan President Museveni implied in his keynote speech to the seminar on the Rights of the Child:

A very bad habit has developed of well-off middle aged people turning to adolescents for sexual gratification. They reason that the youngsters are less likely to have Aids but the adults themselves are often HIV positive although they may not know it (*New Vision*, Nov. 24, 1988).

Although a few countries are considering issuing AIDS education booklets for school children and Uganda has launched full-scale efforts to warn schoolgirls, many parents put up fierce resistance, fearing that such exposure will legitimate premarital sex. Reactions from church leaders have been particularly strong. The Zambian government created a storm of controversy when it published a booklet advising students that those who do not abstain from premarital sex should use condoms (Hilts 1988:31). An organization of religious leaders demanded that the government immediately withdraw the booklet

. . . until a portion dealing with condoms was "suitably amended" (*National Mirror*, April 3, 1988).

But similar reticences arise also from the population at large. A woman complained about the same booklet's frank sexual advice that:

It is not Zambian to talk about sex. Parents never talk to children about sex. Only at marriage, and even then it is the grandmothers and aunts who tell children about it (Hilts 1988:31).

Cultural Barriers to Condoms
and Implications for Heterosexual Relations

Besides the objections raised to giving sexual advice to schoolgirls, further problems arise when the issue of condoms is raised. Certainly the expense of providing African countries with condoms on a reliable basis is prohibitive. As an official in the AIDS Control Program in Uganda stressed,

To condomize the rural areas means money. . . . If you find a man with a torn shirt in the village, it's likely that his condom is torn too (quoted in Watson 1988:34).

But aside from issues of expense and access, condoms raise a fundamental problem: although they generally function well to prevent HIV by keeping the infected sexual fluids of one partner from entering the other partner, they also prevent reproduction. As such, we need to sort out the cultural implications that a woman would invoke if she asked

a man with whom she was cultivating a stable relationship to use a
condom. I will try to stress the cultural logic that shapes Africans' view
of AIDS and condoms, using evidence, when possible, from their quotes.
(Where direct confirmatory quotes are lacking, the conclusions derive
from my background knowledge of analogous situations.)

Cultural Implications of Using Condoms in Africa

Condom Use Denies a Man Children. First and foremost, a woman who
asks her partner to use a condom is preventing him from having children
with her. This obviously troubles African Catholics. Although some
Catholic leaders privately tolerate their parishoners' use of condoms to
prevent AIDS (Hilts 1988:31), on the whole, and certainly in public,
they object vehemently that condoms unnaturally regulate births. But
quite apart from religious objections, the fact that condoms block fertility
makes most people reluctant to use them. In Zambia a man with AIDS
who already had four children was still distraught when he learned
that he should use condoms and thus have no more children (Hilts
1988:30). And one of Schoepf's (in press, p. 15) female respondents
declared,

> . . . if couples begin to use condoms, they will not produce children.
> Children are the goal of marriage. . . . A woman without children is an
> insignificant woman!

Although this wreaks havoc between spouses, it also creates turmoil
among wider kin networks. A perceptive Ugandan physician described
the reaction among families of patients who go home with the disastrous
news of AIDS:

> The doctor would have to tell his patients to avoid sex without a condom
> and not to have children, creating a storm among in-laws and grandparents
> (Hilts 1988:29).

A European psychiatrist working in Zambia generalized about the
problem:

> The most important area of difference between the West and Africa is
> that in the West, people talk about AIDS and sex, about homosexuality,
> about safe sex and sexual release. . . . In Africa, . . . the emphasis here
> is on the impact on the married, the extended family, and the strong
> expectations of family and friends . . . (Hilts 1988:30).

Because of the condom's unavoidable effect on fertility, a frustrated Ugandan author reported that the AIDS issue has lost credibility among Nigerians, where many people suspect that

> . . . the West has finally found a good ploy to force Africans to accept the use of condoms. It claims that condoms should now be used for protection against AIDS, but its real aim is to further its long-term population control plan for Africa (*New Vision*, Dec. 1, 1988).

Since condoms prevent fertility, the policy task of making them acceptable even in urban Africa becomes much more difficult than in areas where most people try to regulate their fertility as a matter of course. An article in the *New Vision* (Uganda, Sept. 14, 1988) summed up the issue:

> Where fertility is seen as proving the virility of men, or as demonstrating the value of women as wives—especially where husbands may discard wives if they do not produce large families—these pressures usually create barriers to family planning, and hence condom acceptance.

That condoms as AIDS prophylactics face an uphill battle in Africa because they limit fertility may not surprise demographers. Less apparent but ultimately more important, I argue, is the extent to which condom use penetrates the core of stable relations between men and women. Because fertility is expected, even demanded, of a viable relationship, a woman who manages to convince a new partner to use a condom initially must soon remove the barrier. By doing so, she signals that she is willing to transform a loose attachment into one she wants to sustain by bearing the man's children. Denying a man children risks a number of things, among them, that he will stop supporting her and find another woman. Consequently, women, as subordinate members of most heterosexual relationships, are unlikely to demand condom use of men they want to keep.

The fact that condoms preclude fertility comprises a cornerstone of people's reluctance to use them, and underlies virtually all the other implications that follow.

Women Who Ask for Condom Use Are Promiscuous/Prostitutes. Because fertility is demanded of stable relationships, people tend to associate condom usage with partners to whom they are only loosely attached, thus reinforcing their image as devices for promiscuous people or prostitutes. A high level health official in Nigeria implied this, arguing that:

. . . because it is not possible to suppress the natural urge [promiscuity] altogether, the use of condoms would be advocated (*New Nigerian*, March 27, 1987).

A woman who asks her partner to use a condom may also be implying that not only is she promiscuous, she is a prostitute—an implication that makes many young women avoid condoms completely (Shoepf, personal communication). Ironically, well publicized efforts to distribute condoms to high risk groups such as prostitutes further reinforce the idea that only people of loose morals use them. Associations of condoms with promiscuity also lead to allegations that because condoms are not failsafe, promoting them may actually increase the spread of AIDS. The Zambian clergy, for example, stated in a booklet entitled "Choose to Live" that:

Giving condoms even to the unmarried is immoral because it condones promiscuity and results in more of the very conduct which today it is necessary above all else to discourage. Even if condoms reduce the risk of contracting AIDS in single actions, when used on a large scale they are likely to increase the incidence of the disease, because the number of acts by which it is spread will be greatly multiplied (quoted in the *National Mirror*, Sept. 3, 1988).

Condom Use Signals a Desire to End a Relationship. Because of fertility's pivotal role in helping women sustain ties to men, a woman who fears that her husband has been conducting outside affairs may be reluctant to ask him to use condoms, lest she signal a wavering commitment to the relationship. Even if she is securely married, refusing to have more children can be grounds for divorce, an act that incurs the wrath not only of her husband and his family but her own family as well.

A Woman Who Uses Condoms May Have an Outside Lover. The reason? Obviously, she is denying her current partner children; but since fertility is so valued, she must want children by someone else—a man with whom she must be having an affair. I would guess, in fact, that a woman insisting on her husband using condoms may open herself to legal charges of adultery. In an analogous incident from Sierra Leone, a young man broke off his relationship with his steady girlfriend when she accidentally spilled the contents of her handbag and revealed a condom. Since she had not been using condoms with him, he suspected her of having an outside boyfriend (H. Borbor Kandeh, personal communication).

Implications of AIDS for
Heterosexual Relations and Condoms

Having established that fertility impairment is the chief disadvantage
to condoms in a region where most of the population is unwilling to
make the fertility transition, we can examine explicitly the impact of
AIDS on people's already-strong reluctance to use condoms.

A Woman Who Requests Condom Use Suspects HIV Infection. Because
of fertility's value, people may infer that only the threat of HIV infection
would make most women dare to ask a man to use a condom. This
inevitably associates condom usage with AIDS. Three important implications follow.

A Woman Who Requests Condom Use May Have HIV. Because people
usually blame women for HIV transmission, a woman who asks her
partner to use a condom may signal that she herself is infected. Requesting
condom use therefore brands a woman not only as disreputable but as
exposed habitually to AIDS risks, as a young Tanzanian man's remarks
suggested:

> . . . girls in fact were not talking of AIDS allegedly because they don't
> want to scare off boys (*Daily News*, Dec. 1, 1988).

*A Woman Who Requests Condom Use Suspects That Her Partner Has
HIV.* Because condom usage is associated with AIDS, and because a
person infected with HIV is branded as promiscuous, a woman who
wants her partner to use a condom accuses him indirectly of consorting
with other women. In doing so, she jeopardizes a stable relationship
and an important source of economic support. A Zairean woman with
four young children described the economic dangers of alienating a
husband thus, and went on to say:

> If a wife were to *suggest* [using condoms] . . . her husband immediately
> would react unfavorably. He would think: "She is accusing me of infidelity!"
> (quoted in Schoepf, in press, p. 15).

A *New Vision* (Sept. 14, 1988) article in Uganda underscored women's
vulnerability on such matters by pointing out that

> . . . even raising the issue [of condoms] for discussion pose [sic] enormous
> problems for women in certain settings: the male partner take [sic] this
> as a sign that he is not trusted to be faithful, or as an admission on the
> part of his partner that she has another lover, and therefore that he may
> be in need of protection against possible infection.

Policy Conclusions

I have attempted to extrapolate from recent African print media some bellweather indicators of how Africans are responding to the AIDS epidemic and to advice for avoiding infection. The policy issues that arise from this synthesis bear relevance for three areas that appear at first glance to be only remotely related, but, in fact, contain important connections to the themes of fertility and promiscuity that emerged above.

The Fate of AIDS Orphans: Children Whose Mothers Die from AIDS

Concerning the effects of AIDS on children, most media attention has been devoted to children who contract HIV in the womb. Yet the disease poses long-term risks for a group that studies of the social and behavioral correlates of AIDS have hardly begun to recognize: the uninfected children of parents who die of AIDS. Spectres of poverty and homelessness for such children are close to home for Ugandans who draw parallels between the current AIDS epidemic and the ordeal of 20 years of recent war that took enormous tolls on families. A commentator pointed out in *New Vision* (Nov. 24, 1988):

> Children are affected because many of them will become orphans. War frequently takes the father but leaves the mother. There are many [war] widows in Luwero bringing up children under very difficult conditions. Aids will take both parents.

In the public media of other countries as well such concerns are beginning to receive considerable attention (see also Obbo 1989). A Zambian policy maker warned that his country

> . . . may be left with old people too frail to till the land and children without parents to fend for them in the towns (*National Mirror*, Aug., 20, 1988).

Even though extended family members frequently take in orphans, they, like other fosters, tend to be excluded first when food and money are scarce. (Chinua Achebe's novel *Arrow of God* [1969:2–3] describes a new moon as being "as thin as an orphan fed grudgingly by a cruel foster-mother.") Hence, young foster children and orphans face more risks of morbidity and mortality than those with mothers present (Bledsoe et al. 1988).

Like orphans, illegitimate children suffer discrimination from caretakers and have lower survival chances than other children (see Adegbola 1988). Yet if being an orphan is compounded by the stigma of suspected illegitimacy, one of the most pernicious results of a woman's death from AIDS is that even her uninfected children may suffer lower chances of survival. As Sierra Leoneans often stressed to me, a man who believes himself to be the children's legitimate father will invest in their care; thus, children's well-being rests heavily on their mothers' perceived sexual morality. This suggests that the children of a woman who dies of AIDS are doubly susceptible to neglect: because the mother is suspected of promiscuity, her previous behavior may come under question, and all her children may be suspected as the products of illicit unions, making their father and his kin repudiate them. A counselor at The AIDS Support Organization in Uganda confirmed this ominous trend:

> If it is the wife who gets sick first, the husband may even disown the kids saying, "They are not mine" (Watson 1988:34).

In general, moreover, how adults treat children generally reflects their own respect for, or obligations to, the parents (Bledsoe, in press, a). Since most people seem to cast a female AIDS victim as promiscuous, they are likely to generalize their contempt toward her children as well, resulting in almost certain discrimination against her children.

Although relatively little on AIDS orphans has appeared in international stories, the African press is beginning to raise important questions about them, especially in the light of national economic difficulties. Where do these children go and who actually takes on the economic burden of raising them? If people fear contamination from them (regardless of their lack of infection), are they sent far upcountry, away from schools, health facilities, etc.? What impacts would such geographical movements of children have on child mortality, labor, and access to medical facilities?

Female Education

Young urban women comprise one of the groups most at risk of contracting HIV. According to the evidence presented here, one subgroup of them—schoolgirls—face yet more risks. What will be the outcome of these new risks for female education in general?

Despite the advantages of education for girls, people worry that schools expose girls to AIDS risks. As a result, parents may grow even more reluctant than ever to send girls to school. This in turn may result in earlier marriage, higher fertility rates, less interest in using birth control devices such as condoms, lower formal sector work for women, and so on. Efforts by families to take their post-pubescent daughters out of school might be compounded by national efforts to encourage women to marry early because of the AIDS crisis. Drawing attention to the exorbitant bridewealth demanded by girls' parents of the girls, Uganda's President Museveni declared:

> We should control parents in some of our societies who sell their children for money; and hence frustrating young people from getting married (*New Vision*, Nov. 11, 1988).

I suspect, however, that most people are so anxious to educate their daughters that they will continue to press for this, although they may enroll them closer to home, in less prestigious schools and under tighter supervision. A recent newspaper report from a Ugandan village reflected this possibility. When villagers began to realize that a number of their daughters were returning from Kampala suffering from advanced cases of AIDS, they regretted allowing their daughters to go to the city:

> They always contracted that killer disease in Kampala, and come back to die here. . . . At the burial of the last victim recently, people were heard to curse the day when their children went to Kampala. Those whose children are still there are trying to retrieve them from there (*New Vision*, June 10, 1988).

Condoms

It is easy to overlook the strength of local beliefs that have redefined technologies that outwardly resemble our own. An important part of this paper has asked, therefore, how condoms, once placed in the African context, seem to have taken on meanings that their advocates in other parts of the world may not appreciate fully.

The fact that the condom necessarily prevent births as well as disease makes it difficult to convince most African women to use them, for they fear alienating their male partners. According to Watson (1988:34), in fact, most AIDS experts in Uganda say condoms are not the answer. To alleviate some objections to condoms, one might advocate the development of innovative condoms: for example, an internal one that women could wear in secret. But as I have argued, in Africa children are necessary to sustain a stable union. Hence, although prostitutes may use them with temporary customers, women are unlikely to ask men with whom they begin to cultivate longer term relations to use condoms. (Schoepf [MS] points out another potentially viable solution: advising women to use condoms for every sexual episode except when conception is sought. As *Projet Connaisida* workers have discovered, however, many

people believe that a fetus grows by repeated acts of intercourse throughout the pregnancy.)

Condoms for AIDS and Birth Control

Although I have argued that African ideologies make people shun
condoms because they curtail fertility and suggest promiscuity, the present
analysis of heterosexual dynamics suggests a certain logic. At the risk
of seeming to contradict much that I said above, secondary schools may
well be the best arenas in which to introduce condoms and AIDS
education in general. This is by no means an original idea. Many African
governments have thought through more of the difficulties that AIDS
education packages entail for schools than I have.[2] Certainly they are
painfully aware of the public outrage that such programs inevitably
arouse. The following discussion simply explicates the sociocultural logic
of the situation, leaving actual policy discussion to others much more
qualified to take it on. This discussion, then, is merely a small vote of
support for those interest groups in some African countries that are
risking enormous unpopularity by trying to push for education on
condom usage in secondary schools.

Why conclude, then, that schoolgirls might be useful targets of more
intensive AIDS education and condom exposure? Demographers might
argue that introducing condoms in schools would waste money and
effort because schoolgirls present considerably fewer statistical risks of
contracting AIDS than, say, prostitutes. To answer this question, therefore,
we should cast the issue in broader terms. Professionals concerned with
AIDS in Africa seem to be falling into two warring camps: those who
minimize the demographic impact of AIDS in the light of continued
high fertility, and those who emphasize the havoc wrought by death
and destruction. Is it possible for one solution to appeal to both factions?
There may be unexpected cultural links between the solutions that both
AIDS and fertility professionals can utilize to their advantage.

The first link is the identification of a likely target group for more
intensive condom education efforts. Although most Africans dislike
condoms because they block fertility, some urbanites—notably schoolgirls—express considerable interest in curtailing their fertility. They
certainly place themselves at risk by attempting illegal abortions. Hence,
schoolgirls, who are considered to be at risk of HIV infection and have
much to lose by getting pregnant and attempting abortion, would likely
be quite receptive to condoms as means to avoid AIDS infection. When
they grew older, this group would be used to condoms. If and when a
fertility transition were to gather significant momentum, they almost
certainly would be in the vanguard of fertility regulators. Identifying

schoolgirls as logical recipients of condoms campaigns has additional appeal in terms of cost effectiveness. Whereas trying to urge the general populace at large to adopt condom usage may have limited impact, schoolgirls represent a concentrated group of high-likelihood recipients.

Second, the very African cultural link itself between condoms and fertility reduction presents a logic that women might be able to exploit in their own relationships. Certainly asking a man to use condoms is difficult under any circumstance. Whether birth control worries or AIDS fears are uppermost in people's minds is hard to say. Some women are obviously more concerned about avoiding pregnancy and others have reason to fear AIDS infection from their partners. Only individual women themselves can sense which rationale for using condoms—AIDS or birth control—will least antagonize their partners, in very specific contexts. Young women may use the excuse of using condoms as an effort to avoid AIDS when they really want to avoid pregnancy. On the other hand, older women who suspect their husbands of infidelity with infected partners may construe their desire to use condoms as an attempt to avoid pregnancy. In some ironic way, therefore, governments' efforts to publicize the AIDS epidemic and the utility of condoms as AIDS prophylactics may do the most service to women by providing them with credible elements of ambiguity and deniability.

Notes

Acknowledgments. A previous version of this paper was presented at the IUSSP Seminar on "Population Policy in Subsaharan Africa: Drawing on International Experience" in Kinshasa, Zaire, Feb. 27–March 2, 1989. I thank Karen Tranberg Hansen, H. Borbor Kandeh, Robert Launay, Henry Mosley, William Murphy, Musufiki Mwanswali, Etienne van de Walle, and Brooke Schoepf for their help and advice on this paper. I alone, however, am responsible for the analysis and conclusions.

1. Although many Africans understand the basic Western scientific explanations for the causes and means of transmission of AIDS, misconceptions inevitably arise. Some people attribute the virus to external influence. Some Ugandan villagers blame the U.S. Central Intelligence Agency for creating the virus (*New Vision*, July 12, 1988). More extreme were the ideas expressed in a letter to the editor of the *New Vision* (Oct. 4, 1988), that the World Health Organization developed the virus and introduced it secretly to Africa through smallpox and hepatitis vaccines to perform annihilation experiments. And as in the U.S., many devout Africans attribute AIDS to devine justice for promiscuity. On the whole, however, ideas about the etiology of AIDS have entered local cultural repertoires for explaining misfortune. AIDS is attributed especially to breaking important cultural rules, as the President of Uganda discovered to his exasperation:

On a trip to Rakai, the worst-affected district, peasants told him that AIDS would go soon because they were now good: They had stopped stealing goats (Watson 1988:32).

2. Parental resistance would unquestionably doom such efforts to failure without strong government support. Besides the objections described above, parents often suspect that male teachers take sexual advantage of their pupils. Hence, they would be outraged if teachers were apparently handed public license to encourage the girls to be more sexually available. Indeed, some parents would probably take their daughters out of school before exposing them to such programs.

References Cited

Achebe, C. 1969. Arrow of God: A Novel of an Old Nigeria and a New Colonialism. Garden City, NY: Anchor Books.

Adegbola, O. 1987. A Comparative Analysis of Children of Informal and Formal Unions. Paper presented at the IUSSP seminar on Mortality and Society in Sub-Saharan Africa. Yaounde, Cameroon.

Ajayi, J.F.A. 1969. Colonialism: an Episode in African History. *In* L.H. Gann and P. Duignan, eds.g, Colonialism in Africa. Cambridge: Cambridge University Press.

Akingba, J.B. 1977. Abortion, Maternity, and Other Health Problems in Nigeria. Nigerian Medical Journal 7:465–71.

Aryee, A.F. and Gaisie, S.K. 1979. Fertility Implications of Contemporary Patterns of Nuptiality in Ghana. *In* L.T. Ruzicka, ed. Nuptiality and Fertility. Proceedings of the IUSSP seminar on Nuptiality and Fertility, January 1979. Bruges, Belgium: Ordina Editions.

Bledsoe, C. 1980. Women and Marriage in Kpelle Society. Stanford: Stanford University Press.

———. In press, a. "No Success without Struggle:" Social Mobility and Hardship for Sierra Leonean Children. Man.

———. In press, b. School Fees and the Marriage Process for Mende Girls in Sierra Leone. *In* Beyond the Second Sex, Peggy Sanday, ed. Philadelphia: University of Pennsylvania Press.

Bledsoe, C., D.C. Ewbank, and U.C. Isiugo-Abanihe. 1988. The Effect of Child Fostering on Feeding Practices and Access to Health Services in Rural Sierra Leone. Social Science and Medicine 27:627–36.

Bongaarts, J. 1988. Modeling the Spread of HIV and the Demographic Impact of AIDS in Africa. Working Paper No. 140 for the Center for Policy Studies, The Population Council, New York.

Brandon, A. and Bledsoe, C. 1988. The Effects of Education and Social Stratification on Marriage and the Transition to Parenthood in Greater Freetown, Sierra Leone. Paper presented at the Workshop on Nuptiality in sub-Saharan Africa: Current Changes and Impact on Fertility, Paris.

Caldwell, J. and Caldwell, P. 1988. Marital Status and Abortion in sub-Saharan Africa. Paper presented at the Workshop on Nuptiality in sub-Saharan Africa: Current Changes and Impact on Fertility, Paris.

Caldwell, J., Caldwell, P. and Quiggin, P. ms. Disaster in An Alternative Civilization: The Social Dimension of AIDS in sub-Saharan Africa. Canberra: Australian National University.

Cherlin, A. and Riley, N.E. 1986. Adolescent Fertility: An Emerging Issue in sub-Saharan Africa. Technical Note 86-23. Technical Note 85-20. Washington, D.C., Population, Health, and Nutrition Department, The World Bank.

Comaroff, J.L. and S. Roberts. 1977. Marriage and Extra-Marital Sexuality: the Dialectics of Legal Change among the Kgatla. Journal of African Law 21.

Evans-Pritchard, E.E. 1951. Kinship and Marriage Among the Nuer. Oxford: Clarendon Press.

Frank, O. 1985. Demand for Fertility Control in sub-Saharan Africa. Technical Note 85-20. Washington, D.C., Population, Health, and Nutrition Department, The World Bank.

Frank, O. and McNicoll, G. 1987. Fertility and Population Policy in Kenya. Population and Development Review 13:209–43.

Goffman, E. 1974. Frame Analysis: An Essay on the Organization of Experience. New York: Harper Colophon Books.

Guyer, J.I. 1988. Changing Nuptiality in a Nigerian Community: Observations from the Field. Paper presented at the IUSSP Workshop on Nuptiality in sub-Saharan Africa: Current Changes and Impact on Fertility, Paris.

Hilts, P.J. 1988. Dispelling Myths about AIDS in Africa. Africa Report, Nov/Dec.

Kulin, H.E. 1988. Adolescent Pregnancy in Africa: A Programmatic Focus. Social Science and Medicine 26:727–35.

Obbo, C. 1989. Women's Autonomy, Children and Kinship. Paper presented at the African Studies Workshop, University of Chicago.

Peel, J.D.Y. 1983. Ijeshas and Nigerians. Cambridge: Cambridge University Press.

Population Reports. 1982. Update on Condoms—Products, Protection, Promotion, Vol. X, No. 5, H-122–H-156.

Schoepf, B.G. MS. Political Economy, Culture and AIDS control.

Schoepf, B.G., Rukarangira, wa N., Walu, E. and Payanzo, N. MS. Action Research on AIDS in Central Africa.

Schoepf, B.G., Rukarangira, wa N., Schoepf, C., Walu, E. and Payanzo, N. 1988. AIDS and society in Central Africa: A View from Zaire. In AIDS in Africa: The Social and Policy Impact. N. Miller and R.C. Rockwell, eds. Washington, D.C.: Edwin Mellen Press.

Schoepf, B.G. In press. Women, AIDS and economic crisis in central Africa. Canadian Journal of African Studies.

van de Walle, E. and Palloni, A. 1987. AIDS in Africa. Paper presented at the IUSSP Seminar on Mortality and Society in Sub-Saharan Africa, Yaounde, Cameroon, to be published in van de Walle, E., Pison, G., and Sala-Diakanda, M., eds. Mortality and Society in Sub-Saharan Africa. London: Oxford University Press (in process).

Watson, C. 1988. An Open Approach to AIDS. Africa Report Nov./Dec.

About the Contributors

Caroline Bledsoe is Associate Professor of Anthropology at Northwestern University. She has conducted field research in Liberia and Sierra Leone on changing marital patterns, child fosterage and mortality, fertility, and development. She has published findings from this research in such journals as *American Ethnologist, Man,* and *Social Science and Medicine,* and she has contributed papers to several edited volumes. Dr. Bledsoe published *Women and Marriage in Kpelle Society* (1980), based on her research in Liberia. Currently, she is working on a book-length manuscript based on her recent research in Sierra Leone.

W. Penn Handwerker is Professor of Anthropology at Humboldt State University on California's north coast. He has conducted field research in West Africa and the West Indies on various aspects of human population ecology, especially the political economy of development. He has edited *Culture and Reproduction: An Anthropological Critique of Demographic Transition Theory* (Westview, 1986) and is the author of *Women's Power and Social Revolution* (1989).

Warren M. Hern is a physician and epidemiologist whose first work in fertility control after medical school began in Brazil during his service as a Peace Corps Physician in 1966-68, and who currently works in fertility control through his private practice. Dr. Hern's varied career has included teaching and studying at the University of North Carolina, where he received an M.P.H. and a Ph.D., field research among the Shipibo Indians of Peru at various times since 1964, serving as Medical Director of a Spanish-language training program in family planning for Latin American physicians and nurse-midwives under contract with the Agency for International Development, and serving as Chief, Program Development and Evaluation Branch in the Family Planning Division, Office of Health Affairs, in the Office of Economic Opportunity in Washington, D.C. In that capacity, he supervised activities in OEO's $24 million Family Planning Program, served on the American Public Health Association Subcommittee on Family Planning Methods, and prepared the OEO Sterilization Guidelines that were suppressed by the Nixon administration. He also initiated a pilot voluntary sterilization program for poor people living in Anderson County, Tennessee and a statewide family planning program in Colorado. In 1972, he resigned his position at OEO in protest of the sterilization guidelines suppression. In 1973, he was invited to help start a private, non-profit abortion clinic in Boulder, Colorado. In January 1975, he opened his private medical practice, Boulder Abortion Clinic, which he operates in Boulder, Colorado. Dr. Hern is the author of 25 professional publications concerning abortion and human fertility, including *Abortion Practice,* a medical textbook published in 1984. He is also the author of numerous articles and editorials published in *The Progressive, The New Republic, The New York Times,* and various other newspapers and magazines.

Rose Jones is a graduate student in the Department of Anthropology at Southern Methodist University whose research interests focus on women, reproduction, and power. She has conducted research on infertility and reproductive technologies in the United States, and currently is carrying out field research on the West Indian island of St. Lucia.

Patricia A. Kaufert is Associate Professor in the Department of Community Health Services, Faculty of Medicine, University of Manitoba. She is a medical sociologist/anthropologist/epidemiologist. Dr. Kaufert's research has always been in the area of women's health, with a particular focus on menopause.

Catherine L. Leone is a demographic anthropologist who is now Visiting Scholar at the Carolina Population Center, University of North Carolina. She has conducted field research in Washington State and North Carolina on women's motivations for reproduction. Dr. Leone's current research contrasts the views of sex, marriage, and motherhood expressed by women who belong to the National Organization for Women and by women who are members of the Roman Catholic Church.

John O'Neil is Assistant Professor of Medical Anthropology in the Department of Community Health Sciences, Faculty of Medicine, University of Manitoba. Twelve years of periodic field research in Canadian Inuit communities on health issues provide a basis for a program of collaborative, participatory research with Inuit organizations on northern health policy problems. He is currently the Canadian coordinator for a new collaborative medical research project in Siberia involving aboriginal peoples from Canada and the U.S.S.R. Other important publications include "The Politics of Health in the Fourth World" *Human Organization* (1986), and "The Social and Political Context of Patient Dissatisfaction" *Medical Anthropology Quarterly* (in press).

Barbara Pillsbury is a medical anthropologist who is the founder and senior partner in the consulting firm International Health and Development, and a Fellow of the U.S.-China Educational Institute. She has taught at UCLA, San Diego State University, and various universities outside the United States. She has conducted fieldwork primarily in Egypt, Taiwan, and Bangladesh, on maternal and child health, family planning, women's issues, and development evaluation. She has served as a consultant for numerous international development agencies including the World Health Organization, UNICEF, USAID, and the International Science and Technology Institute. Dr. Pillsbury has published articles in *Social Science and Medicine* and is the author of several monographs, including *Household and Community Beliefs and Practices that Affect Maternal Health and Nutrition* (1989) and *Reaching the Rural Poor: Traditional Health Practicioners are There Already* (1979.)

Carolyn Sargent is Associate Professor of Anthropology at Southern Methodist University. She has conducted research on gender and reproduction in the People's Republic of Benin and, most recently, in Jamaica. Dr. Sargent is the author of *The Cultural Context of Therapeutic Choice* (1982). Her book *Maternity, Medicine, and Power: Reproductive Decisions in Urban Benin* is forthcoming. Dr.

Sargent, together with Thomas Johnson, is currently editing the text, *Medical Anthropology: A Handbook of Theory and Method.*

Jeanne M. Simonelli is Assistant Professor of Anthropology and Black and Hispanic Studies at the State University of New York campus at Oneonta. Her interest in Hungarian fertility is related to past and present research concerning agriculture, economics, and women's roles in Mexico, Hungary, Oklahoma, and rural New York. Dr. Simonelli is the author of *Two Boys, A Girl, and Enough* (Westview, 1986), based on her research in Mexico. Her photoethnography *Too Wet To Plow: The Family Farm in Transition* will be published in 1989.

Martha C. Ward is Professor of Anthropology and Urban and Regional Studies at the University of New Orleans. She has conducted field research in Micronesia, the Caribbean, and the United States, and is the author of *Them Children: A Study in Language Learning* (1971; 1986), *Poor Women, Powerful Men: America's Great Experiment in Family Planning* (Westview, 1986), and *Nest in the Wind: Adventures in Anthropology on a Tropical Island* (1989). Dr. Ward is now conducting research on sexual decision-making, women in poverty, urban health, and parenting under pressure.